SURROGACY

REVIEW FOR HEALTH MINISTERS OF CURRENT ARRANGEMENTS FOR PAYMENTS AND REGULATION

REPORT OF THE REVIEW TEAM

Margaret Brazier
Professor of Law, University of Manchester

Alastair Campbell
Professor of Ethics in Medicine, University of Bristol

Susan Golombok
Professor of Psychology, City University, London

Presented to Parliament by the Secretary of State for Health by Command of Her Majesty October 1998

Cm 4068 **£10.30**

Contents

FOREWORD

In June 1997, we were asked by the United Kingdom Health Ministers to review certain aspects of surrogacy arrangements. We were invited to review the current law and practice and charged to attempt "to ensure that the law continued to meet public concerns". We now present our findings and recommendations for reform of the law.

We have not found our task any easier than did the Warnock Committee fifteen years ago. Surrogacy involves an intimate and emotional area of human life. Strong and diverse opinions on the ethics and practice of surrogacy exist in our society and have been forcefully expressed to us. We are extremely grateful to all those who gave evidence to us, participated in discussions with us, and those many people who responded so fully and helpfully to our consultation exercise. We know that there will be numbers of them who disagree with our conclusions. We would want to take this opportunity of saying publicly that we have taken careful note of all that has been said to us and deliberated at great length before reaching our ultimate conclusions. Our especial thanks must go to the respondents who spoke, sometimes at personal cost, of their own experiences of surrogacy.

Finally we must thank the staff of the Department of Health who have given us such invaluable support in conducting the Review and preparing this Report. We are particularly grateful to our Secretary, Mr M Evans, Dr E Gadd, whose advice on matters both medical and ethical has enlightened and enlivened our deliberations and to Ms S Ryan who provided invaluable legal advice to us at all times.

Margaret Brazier OBE (Chairman)
Professor of Law, University of Manchester

Alastair Campbell
Professor of Ethics in Medicine, University of Bristol

Susan Golombok
Professor of Psychology, City University, London

August 1998

EXECUTIVE SUMMARY

1. In June 1997 the United Kingdom Health Ministers asked us to examine certain aspects of surrogacy arrangements "to ensure that the law continued to meet public concerns". Our terms of reference required us to consider whether payments, including expenses, should continue to be made to surrogate mothers; whether a recognised body or bodies should regulate such arrangements; and if changes are required as a result to the Surrogacy Arrangements Act 1985 and/or the Human Fertilisation and Embryology Act 1990.

2. In conducting our Review, we have consulted as widely as possible with individuals and organisations with interests in the practice of surrogacy. We considered it to be especially important to obtain the views of people who have actually been involved in surrogacy arrangements. As others have before us, we found substantial difficulty in obtaining hard evidence about the incidence, nature and outcomes of surrogacy arrangements. We believe that a high priority must be accorded to measures which will help to ensure that such information, including information about the welfare of children born as a result of surrogacy arrangements, is more readily available in the future.

3. In the first three chapters of our Report, we outline the context of our Review, revisit the findings of the Warnock Committee on surrogacy, and trace the development of surrogacy from 1984 to the present day. We find that the incomplete implementation of the recommendations of either the majority or the minority of the Warnock Committee created a policy vacuum within which surrogacy has developed in a haphazard fashion.

4. In Chapter 4, we analyse the underlying social, ethical and legal issues inherent in surrogacy arrangements as we perceive them in 1998. We address the psychological implications of surrogacy arrangements, consider how procreative liberty and welfare may be balanced, and examine the role of law in such a personal and intimate area of human life. We conclude that the risks of harm, primarily to the child to be born, but also to the adults involved in surrogacy arrangements, justify a degree of regulation of surrogacy arrangements. We find that payments to surrogate mothers, other than in recompense for genuine expenses, give rise to the following concerns. (1) Payments create a danger that women will give a less than free and fully informed consent to act as a surrogate. (2) Payments risk the commodification of the child to be born. (3) Payments contravene the social norms of our society that, just as bodily parts cannot be sold, nor can such intimate services.

5. Currently there is no direct prohibition preventing payments to surrogate mothers for their services. However, when a commissioning couple apply for a parental order or to adopt the child, it is in theory a bar to the grant of such an order that the surrogate mother has been paid more than expenses. In certain cases, the amounts paid today as "expenses" involve in reality a payment for services. We recommend that payments to surrogate mothers be expressly limited to actual expenses occasioned by the pregnancy, and that expenses be statutorily defined by a new Surrogacy Act.

6. As did the minority of the Warnock Committee, we see a strong case for regulation of surrogacy arrangements to protect the interests of all parties to an arrangement. We recommend that agencies involved in surrogacy arrangements should, as now, operate only on a non-profit making basis, and in addition should have to be registered by the Department of Health. The Department would ensure that any such agency has the requisite expertise to assist in setting up surrogacy arrangements and would monitor the activities of agencies.

7. Surrogacy can never be risk free. We believe that every attempt should be made to minimise the risks of surrogacy. Consequently we propose that the UK Health Departments develop, in consultation with the Human Fertilisation and Embryology Authority and other interested bodies, a Code of Practice to set out minimum standards for surrogacy arrangements. The Code of Practice should confirm that the welfare of the child to be born must be the paramount concern of all those involved in any surrogacy arrangement. It should seek to ensure that the interests of surrogates and commissioning couples are adequately protected and that all parties to an arrangement are clear about their expectations of each other. The Code of Practice would be binding on any surrogacy agency. We also hope that the Code will operate as an advisory code to anyone contemplating being involved in surrogacy, including those who enter into altruistic arrangements with friends or family.

8. After much thought, we concluded that new legislation was ultimately required to implement our proposals. We recommend the enactment of a new Surrogacy Act to ban payments other than expenses, to require the registration of surrogacy agencies and to give statutory force to a Code of Practice. Contravention of the ban on payments to the surrogate other than expenses would result in ineligibility for a parental order. It would become a criminal offence to operate an unregistered surrogacy agency.

9. Finally, we recommend that certain measures be implemented immediately and that, pending legislation, the Department of Health seeks to implement certain of our key proposals on a voluntary basis.

Chapter 1

THE REVIEW

1.1 In June 1997 the UK Health Ministers asked us to examine certain aspects of surrogacy arrangements. This was, in the words of Tessa Jowell, Minister for Public Health, "to ensure that the law continued to meet public concerns".

1.2 Our terms of reference were as follows:

- to consider whether payments, including expenses, to surrogate mothers should continue to be allowed, and if so on what basis;

- to examine whether there is a case for the regulation of surrogacy arrangements through a recognised body or bodies; and if so to advise on the scope and operation of such arrangements;

- in the light of the above to advise whether changes are needed to the Surrogacy Arrangements Act 1985 and/or section 30 of the Human Fertilisation and Embryology Act 1990.

Our remit

1.3 We regarded our role as requiring us first to evaluate the evidence relating to the practice of surrogacy in the UK, and second to examine how far existing legal principles as embodied in the Surrogacy Arrangements Act 1985 and section 30 of the Human Fertilisation and Embryology Act 1990 continue to be adequate and appropriate in 1998.

1.4 The issues surrounding surrogacy sometimes arouse strong emotions and in the course of our work we have been asked to consider a number of issues strictly outside our terms of reference. **It is important that we make clear at the outset that our remit was not to consider all aspects of surrogacy**. The Minister took care in her announcement to say what we should not be concerned with:

> *"We have specifically asked the review team to consider the issue within the context that surrogacy should not be commercialised and that any woman who has a baby as part of a surrogacy arrangement should not be compelled to give it up if she changes her mind. We also want to know whether there is, realistically, any practical way in which surrogacy arrangements could or should be regulated and if so how."*

1.5 In other words, our terms of reference specifically excluded consideration of:

i. commercialisation *ie* that third parties should be able to profit from surrogacy arrangements, and

ii. enforceability of contracts *ie* whether the surrogate mother should be bound by a contractual arrangement to give up her child, or whether the commissioning couple should be similarly bound to make the agreed payment.

Events leading to the review

1.6 In 1984 it appears that opinion within the medical profession largely opposed any professional involvement in surrogacy. However in 1990 the BMA published its report *Surrogacy: Ethical Considerations* which endorsed a degree of professional assistance in establishing a surrogate pregnancy. In 1996 the BMA updated that report in its book *Changing Conceptions of Motherhood: The Practice of Surrogacy in Britain*[1]. In that publication the BMA declared surrogacy to be an "acceptable option of last resort" in certain cases but stressed that "the interests of the potential child must be paramount and the risks to the surrogate mother must be kept to a minimum."

1.7 There was also evidence that clinics offering *in-vitro fertilisation* (IVF) were becoming more involved in surrogacy arrangements. This contributed to the impression that such arrangements were becoming more frequent.

1.8 During 1996 and 1997 a number of cases involving surrogacy arrangements were reported. These cases provoked a substantial but mixed reaction both from the media and the public and demonstrated some of the ways in which surrogacy was developing.

1.9 These included in 1997 a case involving a couple from abroad who sought a surrogacy arrangement in the UK. The media reported in detail the difficulties that arose in this case, and the breakdown in the relationship between the parties involved. What should have been a private arrangement took on the appearance of a public spectacle and cast doubt on the ability of the current arrangements to meet society's legitimate concerns about such cases.

1.10 The arrangements for surrogacy in the USA, in particular its commercial nature, also came into the spotlight early in 1997. The director of a US commercial agency visited the UK to recruit commissioning couples who wished to undertake surrogacy arrangements at

---

1 BMA publications 1996

his agency in the United States. It was reported that the charge to the commissioning couple for this service, including medical and legal expenses and payments to the surrogate mother, amounted to £30,000.

1.11 In another case, a full surrogacy arrangement resulted in the birth of triplets. The children were entrusted to the commissioning couple. This was reported almost entirely positively as an example of surrogacy helping those who otherwise would remain childless.

1.12 Other stories also surfaced, including a case in the USA of a couple who arranged for a surrogate to carry their daughter's fertilised eggs after her death to enable them to become grandparents. In the UK more recently we have heard of a mother carrying a child for her own daughter, and of a daughter carrying a child for her mother.

1.13 In particular, concerns were expressed about the welfare of the child in such arrangements and the apparently increasing levels of payment being offered to surrogate mothers - £13,000 was reported in the media in the case involving the couple from abroad referred to in 1.9 above and even higher figures were reported in other cases. This led to suggestions that surrogacy is, in effect, increasingly practised on a commercial basis.

Background to the current law

1.14 The *Committee of Inquiry into Human Fertilisation and Embryology*, chaired by Baroness Warnock (resulting in the "Warnock Report" 1984[2]) was set up in 1982. The Warnock Committee was asked to examine the ethical implications of developments in human reproduction generally, including surrogacy. The Committee conducted its deliberations against a background of considerable public concern about the potential consequences of rapidly developing advances in reproductive medicine.

1.15 The Government in 1984 only partially accepted the broad conclusions of the Warnock Committee in relation to surrogacy arrangements and Parliament implemented certain of its recommendations in the Surrogacy Arrangements Act 1985 and the Human Fertilisation and Embryology Act 1990. The Government took the view then that, because of the legal, ethical and social problems associated with surrogacy arrangements, they should not be encouraged.

1.16 We revisit the findings in the Warnock Report in the next chapter and discuss the framework within which surrogacy arrangements have developed since 1984 in Chapter 3.

---

2 *Report of the Committee of Inquiry into Human Fertilisation and Embryology* (July 1984 Cmnd. 9314)

The consultation process

1.17 We have previously stated that part of our purpose was to "ensure that the law continued to meet public concerns" (Tessa Jowell, Minister for Public Health, 11 June 1997). We saw our task, first, to examine the background and ethics of surrogacy; second, to look at the law as it applies to such arrangements; and, third, to consider if the legal principles as they stand meet the challenges posed by surrogacy arrangements and continue to enjoy public confidence and support.

1.18 We set out, therefore, to obtain as much factual evidence as we could about the practice of surrogacy in the UK, and abroad; about its development since the Warnock Report; and about the impact of the 1985 and 1990 Acts. The opinions of those who were involved in such arrangements, including those involved in an academic and lay capacity, were also very important.

1.19 A problem we have encountered in the course of the review is the relatively limited amount of hard evidence about the incidence and nature of surrogacy arrangements[3].

1.20 One of the reasons for this is that there is no requirement for data to be collected on surrogacy arrangements generally and, indeed, it would be virtually impossible to do so for private arrangements which involve neither health nor social services. We discuss in this chapter the evidence that is available, as well as the outcome of our discussions with individuals and groups.

Sources of information

1.21 In the course of our review we identified a number of sources of information which we discuss below. It was necessary for us to consider the relevance of all the information we received in the context that much of it was likely to be incomplete or open to question. As we note later, we believe that many surrogacy arrangements may be conducted entirely without contact with the health or social services. These arrangements, usually between family members or friends, are unlikely to become a matter of public record.

1.22 In order to seek the views of as wide a range of people as possible with an interest in surrogacy we met a number of individuals and organisations, and undertook two consultation exercises, one with Guardians *ad litem* (independent specialist social workers) and the other with professionals and the public.

---

3 This, too, was one of the problems faced by the BMA in considering this subject in 1996. Their Report: *Changing Conceptions of Motherhood: The Practice of Surrogacy in Britain* (BMA publications 1996) referred to the limited amount of information available.

1.23 We were also provided by the British Fertility Society with the results of a survey of clinics licensed under the 1990 Act to determine the extent to which such clinics are involved in surrogacy arrangements. This showed, among other things, that of 115 clinics licensed by the Human Fertilisation and Embryology Authority (HFEA), 29 had been involved in surrogacy. In addition, we received figures and details of some 250 arrangements made since 1988 from COTS (Childlessness Overcome Through Surrogacy) and of 16 past and 7 continuing arrangements from SPC (Surrogacy Parenting Centre)[4].

1.24 Our three main sources of official data were (i) records relating to parental orders made under section 30 of the Human Fertilisation and Embryology Act 1990; (ii) records kept by Guardians *ad litem* in connection with parental orders and (iii) figures kept by the HFEA on the number of treatment cycles involving *in vitro* fertilisation performed in surrogacy cases.

Section 30 orders

1.25 Under the terms of the 1990 Act the carrying or surrogate mother who gives birth to a child born as the result of a surrogacy arrangement is the legal mother of that child. The 1990 Act also contains complex provisions relating to the paternity of the child.

1.26 Where the commissioning couple wish to become the child's legal parents they may seek a parental order if they satisfy the conditions of section 30 of the 1990 Act or they may apply to adopt the child(ren) under the terms of the Adoption Act 1976. Any such order made by the court confers parental responsibility on them and extinguishes it in respect of anyone else. A court considering an application for a parental order will be assisted by a detailed written report from a Guardian *ad litem*[5].

1.27 Such proceedings take place in the courts and records are kept about them. Information provided by the Office for National Statistics (and their counterparts in Scotland and Northern Ireland) shows that the number of parental orders granted by the courts since 1995, following the commencement of section 30 on 1 November 1994, is -

---

4 Further information about COTS and SPC can be found at paragraphs 3.30 and 3.31

5 See Local Authority Circular LAC(94)25 which provides detailed guidance on the powers and duties of Local Authorities, Health Authorities and Guardians *ad litem* under the terms of the Parental Orders (Human Fertilisation and Embryology) Regulations 1994.

	1995	1996	1997
England and Wales	47	40	39
Scotland	2	2	3
Northern Ireland	0	0	0

Guardians ad litem

1.28 The role of Guardians *ad litem* is set out in detail in Annex B.

1.29 In July 1997 we sent a questionnaire to all 54 Guardian panel managers in England. This was in order to obtain information for the period 1 August 1996 - 31 July 1997 about surrogacy arrangements in which Guardians had been involved as part of adoption or section 30 proceedings.

1.30 We received 60 responses from Guardians (see Annex B for further information about the number of Guardians in England). Of these, 34 reported that they had been involved in section 30 proceedings involving 39 children in this period (see Annex C for a summary of cases). None had been involved in adoption proceedings following a surrogacy arrangement.

1.31 Of the 39 children born, 8 were genetically related to both of the commissioning parents. Medical involvement was reported in 3 further cases. Thus the large majority of surrogacy arrangements were conducted outside licensed clinics. Payments reported to Guardians ranged from nothing to £12,000, averaging £3,800 where payments were made.

IVF surrogacy cases

1.32 The Human Fertilisation and Embryology Authority also provided us with figures for the number of treatment cycles involving *in vitro* fertilisation (IVF) carried out since 1991 for both surrogacy and non-surrogacy cases -

period	IVF surrogacy cycles	IVF surrogacy pregnancies	IVF surrogacy live births	non-surrogacy IVF cycles
1.8.91-31.12.91	0	0	0	6649
1.1.92-31.12.92	7	1	0	18330
1.1.93-31.12.93	45	8	6	21805
1.1.94-31.12.94	71	16	11	24783
1.1.95-31.12.95	57	13	10	29239
1.1.96-31.3.96 (NB: 3 months)	10	1	1	7859

source: HFEA

Public consultation

1.33 Early in the course of the review, we took the view that in this sensitive and highly personal area of human conduct it was important to conduct a consultation exercise in order to obtain the widest possible base of information.

1.34 It was also clear to us that much of the debate about surrogacy that had taken place was based on poor knowledge of the legal position and the conclusions which underpinned the recommendations of the Warnock Report. We saw one purpose of the consultation exercise as providing information to the professional and lay audience to which it was directed to help enable them to reach informed conclusions on the issues raised by the review and the consultation exercise itself.

1.35 The consultation exercise was announced by the Minister for Public Health[6] and received wide media attention. Copies of the document were sent to professional bodies and individuals with an interest as well as to others who asked for a copy. Requests for copies came from Australia, Japan, the USA, Canada and many European countries. In total more than 600 copies of the document were issued and requests continue to be made for the document as a source of information.

1.36 The document set out the background to the review and the law as it stands. It asked a number of questions, reproduced at Annex D, relating to the terms of reference of the review, and invited comments on these and related issues. 369 responses were received - see Annex H for a list of respondents (excluding those whose responses were marked

---

6 Thursday 9 October 1997

confidential - see paragraph 1.40 below). We were pleased to have received 117 responses from people who had been involved in surrogacy arrangements: 38 from surrogate mothers and 79 from commissioning parents.

1.37 In the course of the consultation exercise it came to our attention that COTS had provided its members with suggested responses to the questions asked, based on the organisation's own response to the review. We understand that COTS did advise members that they should answer the questions in accordance with their own personal views although, perhaps naturally, many used the COTS' response as a template for their own. This was possibly because their views coincided in any event. Nevertheless, not all of these responses simply repeated COTS' views; a significant number provided answers in the light of their own experience of surrogacy.

1.38 In our analysis of the responses we believed that it was important to distinguish between those responses which reflected the views of COTS and its members, and those views expressed by others, whether or not they were personally involved in surrogacy. This was because, even although the consultation was not in any sense a "voting exercise", there was the possibility of a significant number of answers from COTS' members providing a misleading impression of the overall findings, and of general public opinion in relation to surrogacy. This is reflected in discussion of the responses to the consultation exercise throughout this report.

1.39 That is not to say that the responses from COTS' members were in any way considered as less significant than other responses; indeed, they were very helpful and in addition provided an excellent snapshot of surrogacy as it is practised today.

1.40 Of the 369 responses, 122 were identified from COTS members. We did not receive any responses that we could identify as being from any other similar organisation. Of the total number of responses, 79 were marked confidential and 9 partially confidential[7].

1.41 A statistical analysis of the overall response is provided at Annex E1 and of non-COTS' responses at Annex E2. As mentioned above, the consultation was not intended to be a referendum; it elicited a great deal of information from a wide range of people and organisations. It can, however, be seen from the analysis that there was a broad measure of agreement on a number of issues:

---

7 The 281 responses not marked confidential and extracts from the 9 marked partially confidential can be inspected by appointment at the Department of Health, HP4B, Room 423 Wellington House, 133 Waterloo Road, London SE1 8UG

i. that there should not be a ban on all payments to surrogate mothers;

ii. that if payments were made to surrogate mothers then this should include loss of actual earnings;

iii. that legislation should define allowable remuneration and/or relevant expenses;

iv. that, if payable, legislation should define maxima for remuneration and/or expenses;

v. that a body should regulate/monitor surrogacy arrangements; and should approve and regulate surrogacy agencies;

vi. that the law should not restrict agencies further, or ban them altogether, but they should be put on a more formal footing;

vii. that couples should be free to decide whether or not to use the services of a surrogacy agency.

Oral hearings

1.42 We invited a number of people who had responded to the consultation exercise to discuss and expand, in confidence, on their responses. A list of those who attended is at Annex F.

1.43 In addition, we held discussions with Baroness Warnock DBE and with the Chairman, deputy Chairman and officers of the Human Fertilisation and Embryology Authority.

1.44 We also met Mrs Justice Bracewell, an experienced judge of the Family Division (who chaired the Children Act Advisory Committee, which made its final report in June 1997) and who has a particular interest in the issues surrounding surrogacy arrangements. Various matters were discussed. These included issues relating to the making of parental orders under section 30 of the Human Fertilisation and Embryology Act 1990 and the operation of that section in practice, the sanctions available should there be any breach of the requirements of section 30, issues regarding the welfare of the child, matters relating to the kinds and amounts of payments made to the surrogate mother, and the question of whether agencies should be involved in surrogacy arrangements.

1.45 We found these discussions very useful.

Seminar

1.46 On 6 April 1998 we held a seminar in London under *Chatham House Rules*[8]. Those invited to attend (Annex G) represented a wide range of backgrounds with practical, professional and academic interests in surrogacy and related issues. The purpose of the seminar was to discuss the issues raised by the review; the options for change and their implications, based on papers provided to those attending; to ensure that all avenues had been explored; and to act as a sounding board for ideas.

1.47 The discussion took place under the three main headings of the review: (i) regulation of surrogacy arrangements, (ii) payments and (iii) legislative reform. The meeting was a challenging one, with many views and suggestions for change being floated and discussed. We also discussed the implications if no changes were made to the current system.

Conclusion

1.48 We are very grateful to all those who responded to the consultation exercises and who attended the oral hearings or in other ways provided us with comments or advice.

1.49 Finally, we are bound to say that, like the Warnock Committee before us[9], we have found even these limited questions to be very difficult indeed. We have taken the views of a large number and range of people in the course of our review and sought throughout to find an answer which did, in fact, "provide a sensible and sensitive way forward within a framework that inspires public confidence"[10] and one that would be practical. The following chapters describe further the context of our work and our conclusions.

---

8 Under *Chatham House Rules,* in order to facilitate free discussion, information provided for a meeting, and the discussion that takes place, may not be revealed.

9 *Report of the Committee of Inquiry into Human Fertilisation and Embryology* (July 1984 Cmnd. 9314) at paragraph 8.17

10 Tessa Jowell, Minister for Public Health, announcing the review in answer to a Parliamentary Question on Wednesday 11 June 1997 (Hansard vol. 295; col. 478 - 479)

Chapter 2

SURROGACY AND THE WARNOCK REPORT

2.1 In this chapter, we review the analysis of surrogacy offered in the Warnock Report and explore both the divergence of opinion within the Warnock Committee itself and the incomplete implementation of the proposals made in the Warnock Report by the Government of the day.

The Warnock Committee

2.2 The terms of reference for the Warnock Committee were:

"To consider recent and potential developments in medicine and science related to human fertilisation and embryology; to consider what policies and safeguards should be applied, including consideration of the social, ethical and legal implications of these developments; and to make recommendations".

2.3 The Warnock Report said of surrogacy that it was a question which "...presented us with some of the most difficult problems we encountered". The Committee was unable to achieve unanimous agreement on a solution to those problems.

2.4 The majority opinion in the Warnock Report accorded great weight to the moral and social objections voiced in respect of surrogacy arrangements in 1984. The Committee unanimously agreed that surrogacy for convenience alone was "totally ethically unacceptable"[11]. For the majority, even where medical grounds made it impossible, or highly dangerous, for a woman to bear a child herself, the danger of exploitation of another person (the surrogate) appeared to outweigh the potential benefits to the commissioning couple "in almost every case". Treating a surrogate as a means to an end was always liable to moral objection. The majority very firmly expressed their judgment that surrogacy was "positively exploitative when financial interests are involved".

2.5 It appears to us that, although the Warnock Report rehearsed other objections to surrogacy[12], including arguments relating to the welfare of the child and the intrusion of a third party into the marital relationship, the fundamental objection of the majority in Warnock to surrogacy rested on the dangers of exploitation of the surrogate. The majority

---

11 At paragraph 8.17

12 At paragraphs 8.10 to 8.12

acknowledged some potential benefits of surrogacy, the happiness of the commissioning couple, and the good inherent in an act of generosity on the part of the surrogate. Nonetheless, for the majority, those benefits could not outweigh the objection of using surrogates as a means to an end.

2.6 The fears of the majority of the Warnock Committee about exploitation where financial interests are involved in surrogacy arrangements led them to conclude that commercial exploitation of surrogacy should be their primary, although not exclusive, concern. Consequently their Report recommended that legislation be enacted making it a criminal offence to create or operate in the United Kingdom *any* agency whose purposes "...include the recruitment of women for surrogate pregnancy or making arrangements for individuals or couples who wish to utilise the services of a carrying mother". Warnock's recommendations expressly proposed that "such legislation should be wide enough to include both profit and non-profit making organisations" and the actions of "professionals or others who knowingly assist in the establishment of a surrogate pregnancy"[13].

2.7 The effect of the recommendations by the majority in the Warnock Report, had they been implemented in full, would have been to prohibit any third party from involvement in the introduction of potential surrogates to commissioning couples, or in the process of assisting to establish a surrogacy arrangement. It would be irrelevant whether any organisation or individual received payment for their role in setting up the surrogate arrangement. Albeit the majority singled out financial gain as the pre-eminent danger in the context of surrogacy arrangements, they recommended restrictive rules designed to limit the practice of surrogacy as much as possible, short of an absolute ban on surrogacy.

Our view of the Warnock Report

2.8 It is our view that had the recommendations of the majority in the Warnock Report been fully implemented, it would have been unlawful for organisations such as *Childlessness Overcome Through Surrogacy* (COTS) and the *Surrogacy Parenting Centre* (SPC)[14] to operate at all, and it is unlikely that clinics licensed to provide fertility treatment by the HFEA would have been prepared to offer surrogacy services for fear of falling foul of the law. Indeed in para 8.20 of their Report, addressing the issue of legal definitions of motherhood where in full surrogacy the female partner of the commissioning couple would be the genetic mother, the Warnock Committee express the view that full surrogacy would be unlikely to occur

13 At paragraph 8.18

14 There are background notes on the two organisations of which we are aware, COTS and SPC, at paragraphs 3.30 and 3.31

because of the probability that any professional using IVF to establish such a surrogate pregnancy would be committing an offence.

2.9 The majority in Warnock rejected the use of the criminal law to prevent private individuals entering into surrogacy arrangements to "...avoid children being born to mothers subject to the taint of criminality". They did recommend that legislation make it clear beyond any possible doubt that surrogacy agreements are illegal contracts and therefore unenforceable in the courts.

2.10 The majority made no express proposals relating to payments to surrogate mothers. Given that their recommendations (as para 8.20 makes clear) would necessarily have provided that the only means by which the commissioning couple could acquire full and joint parental responsibility for the child would be *via* adoption, the majority would appear to have assumed that adoption laws limiting payments to the birth mother to expenses only would operate to prevent payments to the surrogate constituting a profit to her.

2.11 Our understanding of the recommendations of the majority in Warnock is this: the clear objective of those proposals was to implement a legislative framework which strongly discouraged surrogacy arrangements, made transparent society's disapproval of surrogacy as a practice, and limited resort to surrogacy arrangements to, at most, a handful of instances where a relative or a close friend would agree to act as a surrogate on an altruistic basis.

2.12 It is important to note one proposal the majority in Warnock unequivocally rejected. At para 8.18 the Report says:

> "We have considered whether a limited, non-profit making surrogacy service, subject to licensing and inspection, could have any useful part to play but the majority agreed that the *existence of such a service would in itself encourage the growth of surrogacy*". (emphasis added)

2.13 The majority in Warnock thus expressly rejected regulation of surrogacy services. They equated the state's involvement in such services with an official blessing of surrogacy likely to increase the number of surrogacy arrangements, arrangements they regarded as inherently objectionable.

The minority recommendations in the Warnock Report

2.14 Two members of the Warnock Committee issued a powerful dissent to the Committee's recommendations relating to surrogacy. At the core of the minority's recommendation on surrogacy was their judgment that regulation of surrogacy arrangements was required to protect the interests of all parties involved in such an arrangement.

2.15 Before examining the minority's recommendations for regulation of surrogacy in 1984, it is important to note that the minority's perception of the acceptability of surrogacy as a means of overcoming infertility in certain cases was significantly less condemnatory than that of the majority. They accepted that there are "...rare occasions when surrogacy could be beneficial to people as a last resort". They shared the majority's outright opposition to surrogacy for convenience, but in other cases viewed the question of exploitation of the surrogate, using her as a means to others' ends, as less clear cut.

2.16 The minority equally opposed the creation of a surrogacy "market" in which commercial agencies would operate for profit. They regarded surrogacy arrangements as having the potential to lead to serious problems generating very difficult personal, legal and social issues. In their view, issues raised by surrogacy are analogous to those raised by adoption. Just as there is no place for commercial adoption/fostering agencies, so the minority saw no place for commercial surrogacy agencies.

2.17 The minority's judgment that surrogacy might on occasion be beneficial, although it was beset by problems and analogous to adoption, led them to conclude that in "...the best interests of all concerned...and particularly the best interests of the child that may ensue stringent care and control was necessary". Surrogacy arrangements should be expressly regulated.

2.18 The minority's proposals for regulation included three key recommendations:

(i) The statutory authority to be created to regulate infertility treatment should include the regulation of surrogacy within its terms of reference.

(ii) The authority would be empowered to license non-profit making agencies who wished to assist in making surrogacy arrangements. The minority envisaged that only agencies with experience of child-care issues would be licensed and suggested adoption and fostering agencies might be candidates for licensing.

(iii) Access to a surrogacy agency would only be by referral from a gynaecologist.

2.19 The minority argued strongly that some form of regulation of surrogacy arrangements was essential. Their primary motivation rested on their judgment that, whatever measures were taken to discourage surrogacy, the demand for surrogacy would continue, even grow. Lacking any means of obtaining adequate advice, arrangements would be made without medical or counselling support. "Do-it-yourself" arrangements were perceived by the minority as particularly unsatisfactory. Hence, legislation should make provision to ensure that couples who were determined to resort to surrogacy were able to do so in a manner least likely to result in harm to their own interests, the interests of the surrogate and, most importantly, the interests of any child to be born.

2.20 Related to their proposals on regulation, the minority also proposed that "some form of adoption procedure" be open to commissioning couples to enable them to acquire parental status. That procedure, the minority thought, should not bar payments to the surrogate. They suggested "...most surrogate mothers would expect payment for their services". Finally the minority rejected the view that all surrogacy agreements should be illegal contracts. Courts should be free to consider individual cases on their own merit.

Applying that minority view

2.21 It is perhaps helpful to sum up how it appears to us the minority opinion in Warnock might be applicable to the issues referred to us in this Review of Surrogacy. (1) Payments would be permissible, although no tariff for payments, or express discussion of the line to be drawn between expenses and profits to the surrogate, was included in the dissent. (2) Agencies would be permitted to operate on a non-profitmaking basis licensed by the HFEA or some other regulatory body. (3) As an agency could only assist couples referred to it by a gynaecologist, doctors would play a central role in the control of surrogacy. (4) Some form of parental order would enable commissioning couples to acquire parental status. Couples would not, as the majority envisaged, be able to acquire such status only via adoption. (5) Courts would at least be free to enforce a surrogacy contract, presumably including a power to order the surrogate to surrender the child.

2.22 The minority dissent concludes with their judgment that public opinion on surrogacy in 1984 remained unformed. A final judgment on the ethical and social dimension of surrogacy was not possible. Rather than seeking to suppress surrogacy arrangements the minority asked that "...the door be left slightly ajar so that surrogacy can be more effectively assessed".

2.23 Two fundamental issues appear to us to separate the majority and minority in Warnock. First, for the majority the use of a surrogate is classified as essentially unethical in nearly all cases. The use of the criminal law to ban surrogacy altogether, or ban at least exchange of money between commissioning couples and surrogates is perhaps avoided only because of the potential taint of criminality affecting an innocent child. The minority, in contrast, accept that there are circumstances where surrogacy arrangements are intrinsically ethical, even to be commended. Second, the majority clearly hoped that by stringent measures to outlaw any assistance in creating surrogacy arrangements, surrogacy would wither on the vine. The minority could not share this view, fearing that what would ensue was a growth of surrogacy inadequately controlled and so enhancing the risks of surrogacy to all concerned.

After Warnock

2.24 In the event, the Surrogacy Arrangements Act 1985 and the Human Fertilisation and Embryology Act 1990 (the "1990 Act") embodied in full neither the recommendations of the majority nor the minority in Warnock, and in our judgment the legislative framework which evolved to deal with surrogacy rested on no coherent basis of policy. The 1985 Act, enacted swiftly after publicity surrounding the Baby Cotton case[15], outlawed commercial surrogacy agencies only.

2.25 In a subsequent White Paper *Human Fertilisation and Embryology: A Framework for Legislation* (Cm. 259) the Government rejected both the majority proposals to outlaw *any* third party participation in surrogacy arrangements and the minority proposal to license non-profit making surrogacy agencies and to bring surrogacy arrangements within the jurisdiction of what was to become the HFEA.

2.26 The White Paper did propose that the statutory licensing authority review surrogacy from time to time and report to Parliament; and that regulations under the proposed legislation should permit the Secretary of State to lay regulations to extend the authority's powers to include power to license non-profitmaking surrogacy agencies. In the event, these proposals did not find their way into what became the 1990 Act and so no express obligations were placed on the HFEA.

2.27 In the next Chapter, we discuss developments since the Warnock Report leading to the current law and practice relating to surrogacy.

---

15 See paragraph 3.7

Chapter 3

SURROGACY ARRANGEMENTS: CURRENT LAW AND PRACTICE

Introduction

3.1 In this chapter, we outline briefly how the framework within which surrogacy arrangements have developed in the United Kingdom has evolved since 1985. The partial implementation of the proposals of the majority in Warnock and the last minute insertion of section 30 into the Human Fertilisation and Embryology Act 1990, resulted, we suggest, in the absence of any coherent policy relating to surrogacy. Courts, medical practitioners and organisations seeking to offer help to commissioning couples and surrogates were left to do the best they could in a policy vacuum. For the most part, we restrict our examination of evolving practice to the matters expressly referred to us, that is, payments to surrogates, regulation of agencies, and possible amendment of the Surrogacy Arrangements Act 1985 and/or section 30 of the Human Fertilisation and Embryology Act 1990.

3.2 Neither the majority opinion in Warnock nor the 1985 Act expressly addressed payments to surrogates. The Warnock Report ruled out criminalising such payments, but, as we suggested earlier, may have assumed that adoption laws would operate as a sufficient deterrent to the exchange of substantial payments between couple and surrogate. Section 57 of the Adoption Act 1976 provides that it is not lawful to make or give to any person any *payment or reward* in consideration of the adoption of the child, the grant of any necessary consent in relation to adoption, the handing over of the child with a view to adoption, or the making of arrangements for the adoption of the child. However, section 57(3) grants judges power to authorise payments in appropriate cases.

3.3 In 1984, the British Medical Association had through its Council expressed the view that it would be unethical for doctors to become involved in techniques or procedures leading to surrogate motherhood.

3.4 The position in 1985 might perhaps be summed up thus. Commercial agencies had been outlawed. Couples could obtain joint parental responsibility only by applying to adopt the child. If they paid the surrogate for her services, they risked compromising their chances of adopting the child. If doctors would not assist in establishing a surrogate pregnancy by offering full surrogacy or medically supervised insemination, it might be thought that fewer and fewer couples would resort to surrogacy. Surrogacy (as the majority in Warnock desired) would not be banned, but yet be so beset by difficulty as to be effectively discouraged.

3.5 A number of developments over the ensuing years meant that surrogacy did not largely disappear as might have been anticipated: (1) the courts showed themselves (not unsurprisingly) to be more concerned to secure the future of a particular child, than to maintain strict rules on expenses; (2) late in the day section 30 was inserted in the Human Fertilisation and Embryology Act 1990 providing an alternative to adoption for some commissioning couples; (3) professional opinion on the ethics of doctors becoming involved in surrogacy changed significantly; and (4) at least two voluntary organisations came into existence with the objective of assisting commissioning couples to find surrogates and to help the parties set up and follow through surrogacy arrangements.

The adoption cases

3.6 The first child custody case involving surrogacy had been heard in the United Kingdom in 1978, although not reported until 1985 (*A v C* [1985] FLR 445). Upholding the trial judge's refusal to grant custody of the child to the father and overruling his award of limited access, the Court of Appeal was implacably condemnatory of the surrogacy arrangement, decrying the "irresponsibility" of all involved. However, in *A v C* the surrogate mother of the child (born as a result of insemination with the commissioning father's sperm) wished to keep the child.

3.7 The "Baby Cotton" case (*Re C (A Minor) (Wardship: Surrogacy)* [1985] FLR 846) posed a different challenge for the courts. Prior to the enactment of the Surrogacy Arrangements Act, a US surrogacy agency had set up a commercial surrogacy arrangement providing for payment both to the agency and the surrogate, an arrangement whereby Mrs C agreed to be inseminated by sperm from the husband of a commissioning couple resident outside the United Kingdom. A child was born whom Mrs C was entirely content should be entrusted to the commissioning couple. The local authority intervened and Baby Cotton was made a ward of court. Inquiries suggested that the couple were suitable parents for the child and ultimately Mr Justice Latey ruled that the couple be given care and control of the child and allowed to take the child out of the United Kingdom. The judge declared that his duty was to determine solely what was best for this child. Surrogacy, and the commercial aspects of the arrangement before him raised "...difficult and delicate problems of ethics, morality and social desirability". Those problems were under "active consideration elsewhere".

3.8 In *Re C* no application was made to adopt the child, thus Mr Justice Latey was not required to consider whether payments made to Mrs C breached adoption laws. In 1987 in *Re an Adoption Application ((Surrogacy)* [1987] Fam 81) the same judge was forced to do just that. A couple agreed to pay a surrogate £10,000 to have a child for them. A child was conceived as a result of natural sexual intercourse between the husband and the surrogate.

In the event only £5,000 was paid to the surrogate. The surrogate refused to accept the additional £5,000 as she had made money from a publication about her experience as a surrogate. The child was handed over to the couple. The arrangement was "fully honoured on both sides".

3.9 Mr Justice Latey, on the couple's application to adopt the child, had to determine whether the £5,000 paid to the surrogate constituted an unlawful payment or reward contrary to section 50 of the Adoption Act 1958 (the predecessor of section 57 of the Adoption Act 1976). He ruled that the payments made did not contravene the Adoption Act. They were not made to pay the surrogate for agreeing to the adoption of the child. At the time payments were made to her, the process of adoption was not in the forefront of the parties' minds. They were payments to compensate the surrogate for the inconvenience and expenses of pregnancy. He went on to say that, even were the £5,000 to be regarded as contravening the Adoption Act, he would exercise his power to authorise such payment "retrospectively".

3.10 By the time the application for adoption was made, the child in *Re an Adoption Application* was 2 years 4 months old. He had spent his entire infancy with the commissioning couple who according to all the pre-adoption reports were excellent parents. It is difficult to see how the judge could have done other than grant the adoption order however "creative" his interpretations of the Adoption Act might be perceived to be. The judgment illustrates two key points in our Review. (1) Relying on statutory limitations on payments to surrogates dependent *entirely* on preventing commissioning couples from obtaining parental responsibility for the child cannot succeed. Once a child is settled with the commissioning couple and attached to them, the child's welfare will inevitably be a family court judge's priority. (2) Undefined, expenses can "disguise" an almost limitless and unprovable range of payments. It should perhaps also be noted that it is not reasonable in a common law jurisdiction to expect courts *post facto* to develop regulation of surrogacy practice when Parliament has not done so itself.

Section 30 and Parental Orders

3.11 Where all parties were content to implement their prior surrogacy arrangement, adoption laws in practice offered no impediment to the completion of the arrangement. Payments would be unlikely to prevent the grant of the order and the courts showed themselves disinclined to intervene to upset an arrangement which was successful in the sense that the child had been handed over to the commissioning couple. The couple were subjected to the usual scrutiny imposed on all prospective adopters, but were in the happy position of having a ready-made child to adopt.

3.12 When Parliament first came to debate the Human Fertilisation and Embryology Bill the only specific references to surrogacy were in section 36(1) which inserted a new section 1A into the Surrogacy Arrangements Act 1985 making it clear beyond doubt that surrogacy arrangements were unenforceable; and in section 36(2) clarifying the position that the 1985 Act applies to all forms of surrogacy arrangements. What was to become section 30, making provision for applications for parental orders, was inserted only at the Report Stage of the Bill. A couple whose twins had been born as a result of a full surrogacy arrangement complained to their MP when told by their local authority that they must apply to adopt the children. As the genetic parents of the children they objected most strongly to having to adopt "their children".

3.13 Their disagreement with the local authority resulted in wardship proceedings (*Re W (Minors) (Surrogacy)* [1991] 1 FLR 385). The couple's MP proposed a new clause to the Bill enabling certain commissioning couples to acquire parental responsibility for the child, other than via adoption. The Government supported the proposal and introduced the necessary amendment. Section 30 itself sets out only minimal criteria for grant of a parental order. Much of the detail was left to be dealt with in regulations. Section 30 did not come into force until November 1994.

3.14 For the purposes of our Review, the key provisions of section 30 provide:

(i) The commissioning couple applying for a parental order must be over 18, married and at least one of them must be domiciled in the United Kingdom or the Channel Islands or the Isle of Man.

(ii) At least one of the couple must be genetically related to the child and the pregnancy must have been established either by IVF or GIFT or by artificial insemination, and not by natural intercourse.

(iii) The child must already be living with the couple and consent obtained from the surrogate and the child's legal father. The surrogacy arrangement must have been implemented.

(iv) Most importantly the court must be satisfied that "no money or other benefit (other than for expenses reasonably incurred)" has been paid to the surrogate, *unless authorised by the court.*

3.15 Section 30(9) provided for regulations to be made which modified the adoption legislation in respect of parental orders made under that section. The current regulations are the Parental Orders (Human Fertilisation and Embryology) Regulations 1994 (S.I. 1994 No 2767). Those Regulations apply to applications for parental orders some of the rules relating to applications for adoption orders. Section 30 applications are designated family proceedings and provision is thus made for appointment of a Guardian *ad litem* (see Annex B). An application for a parental order will normally begin in the local Family Proceedings Court (magistrates' court) but can be transferred to the County or High Court. Guardians *ad litem* are required to establish whether or not the requirements set out in section 30 have been complied with and whether there is any reason why a parental order *should not* be made in the light of the welfare of the child principle set out in the Adoption Act, as modified by the Parental Orders Regulations.

3.16 Guardians play a crucial role in ensuring the welfare of a child who is to be subject to a parental order. They are also required in effect to police the requirements in section 30 that no payment other than expenses be made to the surrogate.

3.17 In evidence submitted to us, Guardians expressed great unease about their role. Those concerns focus essentially, in our judgment, on three issues: (1) it is suggested that insufficient weight is given to the welfare of the child; (2) it is contended that guardians lack the necessary powers to do the job entrusted to them in connection with parental orders; and (3) Guardians have a special concern about children's knowledge of their origins. We expand in the next two paragraphs of this chapter on the first two of these concerns. The third point is discussed generally in Chapter 4.

3.18 The amendment of section 6 of the Adoption Act made by the Parental Orders Regulations provides that "first consideration" be given to the welfare of the child. Slightly different language is used elsewhere in guidance on parental orders. It has been argued that inconsistencies in language obscure what at least some Guardians believe to the fundamental principle of legal proceedings in relation to children, that the welfare of the child should be *paramount*. The child's interests should trump all others.

3.19 However the major difficulty confronting Guardians in relation to current provisions for parental orders would appear to us to be practical. By the time a Guardian is appointed, the child is in the care of the commissioning couple. The surrogate has surrendered him or her. Disturbing that arrangement itself has welfare implications for the child. Moreover, in any attempt *retrospectively* to evaluate the surrogacy arrangement to check that it complies with section 30, Guardians have profoundly limited powers. They have no access to information held by the licensed clinics. They cannot conduct police checks on commissioning couples, or indeed even check that at least one of the couple is the genetic parent. In checking payments made, Guardians have access only to such information as the couple choose to provide.

3.20 Evidence from Guardians suggests widely differing levels of payments to surrogates. Such diversity, on the evidence presented to the courts, does not appear to be justified by particular circumstances. Payments for the service provided by the surrogate, in excess of any reasonable level of actual expenses incurred as a result of the pregnancy, are currently being made. The nature of section 30 orders which come into play only once the child is resident with the applicants means that there is little courts or Guardians can do to ensure that no unlawful payments have been made.

Changing professional opinion

3.21 In 1984, it appeared that opinion within the medical profession veered against professional involvement in surrogacy and that had the majority proposals in Warnock been implemented, professionals might well have had grounds to fear that any such involvement might be unlawful. By 1990, it was clear that the bar on any third party involvement in surrogacy arrangements would not be implemented, and the BMA had altered its stance significantly from opposition to surrogacy to acceptance that professional involvement in surrogacy might, in appropriate circumstances, be ethical.

3.22 In its 1996 publication *Changing Conceptions of Motherhood*[16] the BMA reviewed the practice of surrogacy in Britain. In its guidelines to health professionals endorsing surrogacy as an acceptable option of last resort, the BMA sets out guidance designed to safeguard the welfare of any child to be born and to minimise risks to surrogate mothers. By 1996, it was also clear that a number of clinics licensed by the Human Fertilisation and Embryology Authority (HFEA) had begun to offer full surrogacy services, and, much less frequently, medically supervised insemination.

3.23 It is necessary to be clear as to just what level of medical professional involvement in surrogacy is now practised and endorsed by the BMA. Care of the surrogate once there is an established pregnancy was of course never condemned. Indeed it would be unethical not to provide such care. In recent years however doctors have been asked both to provide advice on surrogacy and to provide treatment services. Generally such treatment services, if they involve IVF or use of stored sperm, must be provided in a licensed clinic. There are, however, accounts of general practitioners assisting in insemination with fresh sperm.

---

16 See paragraph 1.6

3.24 Where treatment services to establish pregnancy in the surrogate are provided in a licensed clinic, the clinic is subject to the Code of Practice promulgated by the HFEA and approved by the Secretary of State for Health. The HFEA in its Code stresses that surrogacy should be considered only where it is "physically impossible or highly undesirable for medical reasons" for the commissioning mother to carry the child[17]. Where the intending mother has no uterus, or has suffered from habitual miscarriage, or suffers from a medical condition rendering pregnancy a grave risk to her life or permanent health, such criteria would appear to be met. Evidence has been given to us suggesting that, additionally, surrogacy might be contemplated where the intending mother had undergone a series of failed IVF cycles. Establishing a pregnancy in a healthy and provenly fertile surrogate might be perceived as preferable to continued attempts at IVF. Whether such cases constitute use of surrogacy as "a last resort" where pregnancy is impossible may be open to question.

3.25 The Code lays down procedures in relation to the welfare of the child. Clinics offering treatment services in relation to surrogacy stress (in evidence to us) that over and above what the Code of Practice demands, every effort is made to secure the welfare of the child to be born, and to ensure that all parties to the arrangement understand the implications of what they are agreeing to do.

3.26 The change in attitude within the medical profession has had two significant results. "Medical endorsement" of surrogacy adds to its respectability. Couples who wish to utilise full surrogacy where they are the genetic parents of the child can obtain assistance in establishing a pregnancy *via* IVF at a licensed clinic. Couples who seek partial surrogacy but with the reassurance of medical supervision can also do so. In both cases that ability to seek professional involvement is likely to be dependent on ability to pay. There have been to our knowledge at least two instances of health authorities being asked to pay for surrogacy services, but generally such services are confined to the private sector.

3.27 What medical practitioners do *not* involve themselves in, however, is the process by which commissioning couples find a surrogate. Doctors may often now be willing to advise generally on surrogacy arrangements and assist in establishing a pregnancy. They do not (and might well fall foul of the 1985 Act if they did) assist couples to establish a surrogacy arrangement. A couple seeking medical assistance to establish a pregnancy must either have found their own prospective surrogate independently, or have obtained assistance from one of the non profit-making organisations set up to support commissioning couples and

---

[17] *Human Fertilisation and Embryology Authority: Code of Practice* (4th edition - July 1998) at paragraph 3.20. The BMA in its booklet *Changing Conceptions of Motherhood* maintains that surrogacy should only be considered where it is "impossible or highly undesirable" for the commissioning mother to carry a child.

surrogates, such as COTS and SPC (see paragraphs 3.30 and 3.31 below). We understand that some clinics will refer patients contemplating surrogacy to such organisations.

3.28 Other professionals, outside the medical profession, may also now have some professional involvement in surrogacy. Lawyers may be instructed to draw up an agreement between the parties, albeit such agreements cannot constitute legally enforceable contracts. Counsellors may be engaged to counsel couples and/or surrogates. Several professionals may be involved in the consequences of surrogacy arrangements. All are likely to be paid by the commissioning couple and may perceive their primary responsibility as being to that couple.

Surrogacy Groups

3.29 Section 2 of the Surrogacy Arrangements Act 1985 prohibited any person from assisting in the making of a surrogacy arrangement on a commercial basis, thus preventing commercial "agencies" from operating to assist in the creation of surrogacy arrangements. Since 1985, to our knowledge, at least two non-commercial organisations have been set up to assist potential commissioning couples and surrogates to meet each other, enter into surrogate arrangements and to provide support to all parties in such arrangements.

3.30 The better known organisation *Childlessness Overcome Through Surrogacy* (COTS) was set up by a partnership between Kim Cotton, who has herself been a surrogate on two occasions, and Gena Dodd, a commissioning mother[18]. COTS is a voluntary organisation for couples seeking to have a child using surrogacy, and for women prepared to become surrogate mothers. It was established in March 1988 and has grown from 70 members to over 800. It claims to have been involved in about 250 surrogate births. A subsidiary group of COTS, known as *TRIANGLE*, introduces infertile couples to women prepared to become surrogate mothers.

3.31 The second organisation, the *Surrogate Parenting Centre* (SPC), was set up in 1993 by Claire Austin, a former surrogate mother. SPC is a much smaller organisation than COTS, and claims to have been involved in 16 surrogate births. A subsidiary of SPC, *HOPE*, provides the initial contact between prospective commissioning couples and surrogate mothers.

3.32 Self-evidently no organisation involved in assisting in the creation of surrogacy arrangements can charge for their services. They cannot operate a commercial service, and, lacking charitable status and/or links with other established child care agencies, may have

---

18 See COTS Booklet 1997: *Introducing COTS*

difficulty in obtaining the requisite professional expertise and experience. Such organisations operate entirely unregulated at present. On occasion critical comment has been made of their processes for screening surrogates and couples. Emphasis sometimes seems to be placed on the primacy of honouring the arrangement of handing over the child to the commissioning couple[19].

3.33 The Chairman and one other member of COTS, and the founder of SPC, gave evidence to us at our request. Initial costs for membership of COTS amount to £200, and £25 per year thereafter. COTS literature[20] recommends payment of expenses to surrogates including £50 per monthly insemination at home; £100 per embryo transfer or insemination at a clinic without drugs, and £150 with drugs. Other expenses recommended by COTS include loss of actual and potential earnings, maternity clothes, food, travel, child minding, medical and psychological expenses as well as solicitor's costs together with life insurance payments. The literature we received from SPC did not include figures for membership costs or recommended levels of payments for surrogacy arrangements, although they recommend payments for expenses to include travel costs, phone calls, maternity clothes, diet, compensation for time off work, inconvenience, baby sitters and life insurance.

3.34 The view from COTS is straightforward. They would welcome regulation. They would like to be "licensed" to assist in surrogacy arrangements. They are concerned about underground surrogacy, and worried that many arrangements are made without any advice or support, or on the basis of advice from individuals or organisations of questionable integrity. COTS are however equally clear on other issues pertinent to our Review. Surrogates should be paid for their services over and above expenses (about £10,000 to £15,000). Contracts should be enforceable so that a surrogate contracting for payment to enter into an arrangement would be required to honour that contract and hand over the child. COTS express disquiet about the evolution of practice which has allowed surrogacy to grow in the United Kingdom without any form of effective regulation and undirected by any coherent policy. Their preferred solution is a regulated commercial market.

3.35 SPC were also concerned about arrangements being made without advice or support and about the effect such arrangements have on the children involved. In their experience,

---

19 COTS Booklet 1997, *Information for Surrogates*: "Finally and most importantly it would be the final blow for your parents-to-be if you kept the child. You would have robbed them of all hope they have placed in you. You have your own children to go home to, they are empty handed. It is a tremendous trust that your couple have placed on your shoulders......DO NOT BETRAY THAT TRUST." (original emphasis)

20 *Surrogate and Couple Memorandum for Host/Straight Surrogacy*: COTS

those arrangements made between friends and family were most likely to be successful. Arrangements between surrogates and commissioning couples who are not known to them are, in SPC's view, based on a "forced friendship" with underlying tensions. Without successful counselling this often led to bad feelings in the relationship.

3.36 Also, while SPC viewed surrogacy as another form of infertility treatment similar to treatments such as IVF, they were concerned about surrogacy becoming a "cheaper option" than IVF. In particular they were concerned about the possibility of clinics offering surrogacy simply as an alternative to IVF. They thought that, in the light of what they perceived as increasing infertility with a corresponding increase in the number of people approaching fertility clinics, the possibility of surrogacy being offered as an alternative to IVF was likely to increase and this was likely to lead to more cases going wrong.

"Unsuccessful" surrogacy arrangements

3.37 So far in this chapter in looking at the adoption cases and parental orders, we have focused on arrangements where in one sense the arrangement has been successful in that the child has been handed over to the commissioning couple. Publicity about surrogacy has often centred on "unsuccessful" arrangements where the surrogate refuses to hand over the child. The law is clear. A commissioning couple cannot apply for a parental order unless the child is already in their care with the consent of the surrogate. Should they apply for a residence order in respect of the child or try to invoke any other form of legal process to compel the surrogate to hand over the child, they are almost inevitably bound to fail. Surrogacy arrangements will not be enforced by the back door. Unless the surrogate is, quite apart from the surrogacy arrangement, entirely unfit to parent the child, she is unlikely to be ordered to give up the child.

3.38 Such evidence as we have been able to obtain suggests that only in a handful of cases (perhaps 4-5% of surrogacy arrangements) does the surrogate refuse to hand over the child. We are aware that this evidence is partial, being based only on figures from COTS and estimates of contested cases in comparison to the grant of parental orders. The small number of "unsuccessful" surrogacy arrangements does not in any sense minimise the acute pain such circumstances must generate. The commissioning couple's hopes are dashed; they will feel deprived of "their" child. The surrogate and her family will find themselves responsible for a child not planned to be part of that family. The welfare of the child, who may in infancy be the subject of protracted legal proceedings, and later come to know of the disputed custody and separation from his or her genetic parent(s), must be a matter of concern.

A European perspective

3.39 In examining the development of surrogacy since 1985, it is important to note developments elsewhere in the European Union. There is (again incomplete) evidence of a growing number of commissioning couples from other countries seeking to find a surrogate in the United Kingdom. Transnational surrogacy arrangements pose special difficulties. Linguistic and cultural differences may impair understanding between the couple and the potential surrogate. Enlightening the child in later years on his or her origins may be more problematic. Couples with no connection with the United Kingdom cannot apply for a parental order. Agencies concerned with the welfare of the child may be unable to ensure that after the child is entrusted to the commissioning couple, adequate measures will be taken to ensure his or her legal status in the family once abroad.

3.40 The European Commission set up a working party chaired by the moral philosopher, Jonathan Glover, to examine the ethical, social and medical problems generated by the new reproductive technologies. The working party's report was published in 1989[21]. The Glover Report endorsed a restrictive approach to surrogacy in the interests of protecting surrogates from exploitation and children from harmfully prolonged battles between the surrogate and the commissioning parents. Commercial agencies should be prohibited, and the surrogate should not be contractually bound to hand over the child. Payments beyond expenses were to be discouraged.

3.41 However the Glover Report did not seek to exclude the establishment of "public" agencies to assist in surrogacy where clear medical reasons prevented the commissioning mother from bearing a child herself. Nor, though payments to surrogate should be discouraged, did the Glover Report propose that such payments be illegal.

3.42 In the event, the prevailing legislative policy in the majority of European Union states is to impose substantial restrictions on surrogacy. A number of states including Austria, Germany, and Sweden[22] prohibit surrogacy entirely. It is a criminal offence to arrange for a woman to conceive and carry a child to be surrendered to another couple or individual, however that pregnancy is established. Other European Union States, including France, Denmark and the Netherlands prohibit any payment in relation to surrogacy.

---

21 *Fertility and the Family*: The Glover Report on Reproduction Technologies to the European Commission (Fourth Estates, London, 1989)

22 Similarly restrictive legislation has been enacted in Norway.

3.43 Restrictive laws on surrogacy in other countries may well result in couples seeking assistance in the United Kingdom. The ability to pay the surrogate (if in the form of disguised expenses), the willingness of clinics to offer treatment services to establish pregnancies, and the existence of organisations that will help arrange an introduction to a possible surrogate mother, all offer inducements to couples to seek surrogacy in the United Kingdom. We note that COTS' concern about transnational arrangements has led them to decide that:

> "due to legal and administrative costs [COTS] cannot accept couples from abroad unless they reside in Britain for the duration of the arrangement or they have their own surrogate".[23]

Conclusion

3.44 Surrogacy has not "withered on the vine". Since there is no requirement to compile accurate records of all surrogacy arrangements we have not been able to verify or quantify the number of such arrangements. Nonetheless, the evidence available to us suggests that numbers are rising and are likely to continue to do so. Attitudes within the medical profession have changed and professional involvement in surrogacy might, in appropriate circumstances, be considered ethical.

3.45 Current legislative provisions limiting payments to expenses only are ineffective. "Regulation" dependent on retrospective examination of the initial surrogacy arrangement simply does not work. Organisations involved in promoting surrogacy have emerged and information about their operation is far from comprehensive. The majority of European States impose substantial restrictions on surrogacy which may well result in couples seeking assistance in the United Kingdom.

---

[23] SPC, by contrast, say that they "work ever more closely with overseas clinics due to English restrictions on egg donation and surrogacy".

Chapter 4

SURROGACY: SOCIAL, ETHICAL AND LEGAL ISSUES

4.1 In this chapter we review the social, ethical and legal dimensions of surrogacy arrangements in the United Kingdom. Our analysis necessarily revisits some of the arguments rehearsed in the Warnock and Glover Reports but seeks to do so in the context of what we have learned about surrogacy practice both in the past fourteen years since Warnock and from the submissions and evidence presented to us. We focus primarily on the very specific questions referred to us by Ministers. We do not attempt a comprehensive analysis of every aspect of surrogacy.

4.2 As we have already noted, the Warnock Committee unanimously condemned surrogacy for convenience and the majority regarded surrogacy as intrinsically objectionable in almost every case. The Report thus sought to use the law to discourage surrogacy by outlawing any third party assistance in the creation of surrogacy arrangements.

4.3 The Warnock Report referred to the following arguments against surrogacy: (i) it constituted an attack on the value of the marital relationship by the intrusion of a third party into the process of procreation, in a more personal and intimate way than would be the case with gamete or embryo donation; (ii) the use of a woman's uterus for financial profit, as an incubator for someone else's child, was inconsistent with human dignity; (iii) surrogacy distorted the relationship between mother and child, and might be psychologically damaging to the child, or degrading to the child, when it was treated as a commodity in a financial transaction; and (iv) since pregnancy carries risk, no woman should be asked to undertake it for another, in order to earn money.

4.4 The Report then briefly rehearsed some arguments in support of surrogacy: (i) those who regarded it as an intrusion into the marriage relationship need not seek the treatment for themselves, but should not try to prevent others from doing so; (ii) surrogacy need not be seen as a degrading use of a woman's body or as commodifying the child, but rather as "a deliberate and thoughtful act of generosity on the part of one woman to another" (paragraph 8.12); (iii) psychological risks to the child (such as separation from the birth mother) were hard to calculate, and in any case some of these risks were already accepted in the case of adoption; and (iv) women had a right to enter into surrogate relationships if they wished, and there was no reason to suppose that they did so lightly, or that payment compromised the voluntary nature of a woman's agreement to enter into a surrogacy arrangement.

4.5 In the course of our review many of the arguments debated in the Warnock Report were raised again with us. The emphasis of debate has nonetheless changed somewhat. Opposition to surrogacy on the grounds of the intrusion of a third party into the marriage relationship was voiced to us, but only by a very small minority of respondents. Couples whose faith or philosophy requires acceptance of the exclusivity of that marriage relationship perhaps now accept that while their private morality excludes surrogacy for themselves such private choices should not dictate public policy. Indeed across a wide spectrum of opinion, we judge that the existence of surrogacy is now accepted, and that the crucial issue is how far the state should intervene to protect the interests of the parties.

4.6 In 1998, the principal concerns relating to surrogacy appear to be these: (i) does existing law and practice adequately safeguard the welfare of the child? (ii) does, and indeed should, existing law and practice protect the interests of the surrogate, her family and the commissioning couple? While there is unanimous agreement that the law must protect children, there was lively debate about how far if at all the state should intervene to limit the choices of the adult parties to surrogacy; and (iii) is payment to the surrogate for her services acceptable? Do payments contravene ethical values and may payments add to the risks of surrogacy?

4.7 At the time of the Warnock Report, very strong concerns were voiced about the prospect of surrogacy for convenience. A scenario where wealthy career women simply wished to avoid the inconvenience of pregnancy and "employed" others to bear children for them was envisaged. We have seen no evidence of such practices. When a woman has no uterus, or suffers from a condition rendering pregnancy dangerous to her health, it is readily seen that these are compelling medical reasons to consider resort to surrogacy. Surrogacy is a last resort. We have, however, been made aware that where a couple has undergone a number of failed IVF cycles surrogacy may be considered even though pregnancy is not absolutely impossible for the commissioning woman. At what point surrogacy becomes an acceptable alternative to other infertility treatment is now a live issue.

Social and Psychological Issues

Surrogacy and the welfare of the child

4.8 Families created by surrogacy differ from the traditional family in two important ways. (1) The gestational mother and the social mother are not the same. Although this is also true of adoption, surrogacy differs from adoption in that the pregnancy was created with the deliberate intention of the surrogate mother handing over the child to the commissioning couple. (2) In the case of partial surrogacy, the child is genetically unrelated to the commissioning mother, and where a donated embryo is used, the child is genetically unrelated to both commissioning parents.

4.9 No systematic information exists about the long-term psychological consequences for children born as a result of a surrogacy arrangement. To the extent that the experiences of adopted children are relevant to children conceived by surrogacy, it is important to note that adopted children do tend to show a greater incidence of emotional and behavioural problems in comparison with their non-adopted counterparts. Not all adopted children experience difficulties, however. It seems that psychological problems are most likely to occur in adoptive families where the quality of parenting is poor, and where the parents do not communicate openly about the adoption to the child. It is also of relevance that the younger children are at the time of the adoption, the less they are at risk.

4.10 There is a growing body of research on the psychological development of children conceived by assisted reproduction suggesting that the quality of parenting in such families is good and that the children themselves are functioning well, whether or not donated gametes had been used in the child's conception. In so far as surrogacy sometimes involves the use of IVF, and children born as a result of a surrogacy arrangement often lack a genetic link with their commissioning mother and occasionally with their commissioning father as well, these findings can be extrapolated to families created through surrogacy. However, only pre-adolescent children conceived by assisted reproduction have been studied as yet, and their psychological well-being in adolescence and beyond remains unknown. It is at adolescence that issues of identity become salient for children and it is also at adolescence that difficulties in parent-child relationships are most likely to occur.

4.11 It was inevitable that our review was conducted in the absence of empirical data on what happens to children born as a result of a surrogacy arrangement, and we have had to rely instead on knowledge about children in adoptive and assisted reproduction families. Although this body of research indicates that we should not necessarily expect children born as a result of a surrogacy arrangement to be at risk for psychological problems, children born through surrogacy differ from adopted and assisted reproduction children in ways that may be detrimental to their emotional well-being as they grow up. It is not known, for example, how a child will feel about having been created for the purpose of being given away to other parents or, if the surrogate mother remains in contact with the family, what the impact of two mothers will be on his or her social, emotional and identity development through childhood and into adult life, particularly in families where the surrogate mother is also the genetic mother of the child.

4.12 Evidence that we have obtained in the course of this review indicates that it is not unusual for the surrogate mother to remain in contact with the commissioning couple and the child, a situation akin to open adoption whereby the biological mother remains in contact with the adoptive family. Although greater openness is generally believed to be of benefit to adopted children, the direct involvement of the biological mother in the adoptive family remains controversial, with some critics arguing that this could interfere with the security of the child's relationship with the adoptive parents. It is difficult to extrapolate from the experience of open adoption to surrogacy, as children involved in open adoption arrangements had often developed a close relationship with their biological mother before making the transition to an adoptive family.

4.13 Although it might be expected that contact with their surrogate mother would be a positive experience for children in that they could develop a clear understanding of their origins, it remains possible that the involvement of the surrogate mother may be distressing for children and undermine the relationship between the commissioning parents and the child. This may be particularly so where one or both commissioning parents lack a genetic link with the child.

4.14 A further distinction between many children born as a result of a surrogacy arrangement and children who are adopted or born as a consequence of some other form of assisted reproduction is the payment to the surrogate mother. The effect on a child, especially an older child, of learning that the woman who bore him or her was paid to do so is difficult to predict. Particularly in cases where children have a hostile or distant relationship with the commissioning couple, the knowledge that they had been brought into the world as a result of a commercial arrangement may not only have a damaging effect on family relationships but may also interfere with the child's development of a secure sense of identity and positive self-esteem. Furthermore, children who discover that their surrogate mother has had other children as part of a surrogacy arrangement may find this information particularly difficult to accept.

4.15 We are very much aware that the child born in consequence of a particular surrogacy arrangement is often not the only child at risk of psychological harm. It appears that those involved in surrogacy practice strongly recommend that the surrogate should have her own children. We are concerned (as were many of our respondents actively engaged in child welfare) about the impact on the emotional security of these children of seeing their mother give up a sibling, especially for payment, and in some instances on more than one occasion. Awareness of a potential effect on the surrogate's own children is demonstrated by advice from COTS[24] that:

> "We believe it is unfair on your own children for them to actually see the baby you will be giving up, as this makes it all too real for them and could cause problems later. If you intend to continue the friendship...wait until your own children have settled down before you all meet again. If this is unavoidable do ensure that you are not holding the baby but the couple are when your children visit."

4.16 We find ourselves lacking direct evidence of the impact of surrogacy on the psychological welfare of children born as a result of surrogacy and the surrogate's own children. We judge, nonetheless, that there is clear potential of risk to the welfare of such children. Research to identify and quantify that risk is needed urgently. The paramount importance of the welfare of the child is such that we believe that in making judgments about the regulation of surrogacy, the state must act on the precautionary principle. Society has a duty to minimise any such potential risk.

Surrogacy and the interests of adults

4.17 Just as information is lacking on the outcomes of surrogacy for children, relatively little is known about the consequences for the adults involved in a surrogacy arrangement. Although studies of mothers who give up their babies for adoption have shown that this can be an extremely upsetting experience that remains with them throughout their lives, it is possible that relinquishing a child in the context of a surrogacy arrangement may be less traumatic. A study by Eric Blyth of a small volunteer sample of surrogate mothers recruited through COTS suggests that parting with the child can be difficult but that distress can be accompanied by feelings of satisfaction and happiness for the commissioning couple[25]. The long-term effects of being a surrogate mother, and whether there are differences in outcome between surrogate mothers who are genetically related to the child and those who are not, remain unknown.

4.18 In the course of our Review, we did receive accounts of women who suffered distress as a result of entering into a surrogacy arrangement. They felt pressured at times to make decisions they regretted and considered that on occasion they were treated in a demeaning way by the commissioning couple. We know of at least two instances where such distress caused the surrogate to decide to keep the child.

---

24 COTS Booklet 1997: *Surrogate's Information*.

25 "I wanted to be interesting. I wanted to be able to say 'I've done something interesting with my life'": interviews with surrogate mothers in Britain *Journal of Reproductive and Infant Psychology* Vol 12 pp 189-198 (1994).

4.19 It may be argued that adults who choose to be surrogates must, like everyone else, sometimes make hard choices. Risk of emotional or psychological harm is a factor for the surrogate to weigh when agreeing to enter into an arrangement. We are concerned, however, that women may be entering into surrogacy arrangements without full awareness of the physical and psychological risks. Payments may operate as an inducement to enter into surrogacy for women suffering financial hardship. There is evidence that the majority of surrogates are significantly poorer than commissioning couples and have relatively low educational attainments. A number are unemployed, unsupported by a partner and responsible for children of their own. "Professional" surrogacy may appear to be an attractive option for women in these circumstances. Some women clearly regret taking up that option. We regard it as proper that society seeks to implement measures to ensure that nobody enters into a surrogacy arrangement unaware of its possible risks or motivated principally by financial need.

4.20 The impact on the commissioning couple of having a child through surrogacy is also unknown. Parents of children conceived by assisted reproduction appear to be well-adjusted and have stable marriages, at least in the early years of the child's life. In the case of surrogacy, however, a third party is directly involved until the child is born and may remain in touch with the family as the child grows up. It is possible that the involvement of a third party may have a negative effect on the couple's relationship, and on the woman's security in her mothering role, particularly in families where the surrogate mother and the commissioning father are the genetic parents of the child. The only available information on this issue comes from Eric Blyth's study which indicates that difficulties can sometimes arise in the relationship between the surrogate mother and the commissioning couple[26].

4.21 It was strongly argued before us that only the welfare of the child could justify intervention to limit private choices. We concluded that the especial vulnerability of adults in the uncharted waters of surrogacy does justify some degree of state intervention primarily to ensure that all involved do so freely and on the basis of full and accurate information. We are also aware that in raising a family the welfare of adults cannot entirely be divorced from the welfare of their offspring. Psychological harm suffered by the parents may adversely affect children. For example, the effects on a surrogate of giving up the child may have negative consequences for her own existing children. Or a commissioning mother made insecure by continuing contact with the surrogate may find it more difficult to parent the child.

---

26 "'Not a Primrose Path': commissioning parents' experiences of surrogacy arrangements in Britain" *Journal of Reproductive and Infant Psychology* Vol 13 pp 185-196 (1995)

The ethical debate

4.22 Since the publication of the Warnock Report there has been continuing controversy and debate both regarding the arguments used in the Report and the practical conclusions of the majority. In order for us to make our recommendations within our Terms of Reference we have had to revisit the debate as a whole, even although our remit is much narrower than that given to the Warnock Committee of Enquiry. In addressing the ethics of surrogacy, we consider, first, whether the principal argument given by Warnock, that surrogacy is an unwarranted use of a person as a mere means to an end, is decisive. We then discuss some of the other arguments for and against surrogacy, referred to in the Report but not used when it reached its conclusions: the risks to the child, including psychological trauma and commodification; the limits of procreative rights; and the moral character of the surrogacy relationship.

Exploitation

4.23 Is a surrogacy arrangement potentially exploitative of the surrogate mother, and positively so when financial interests are involved? The Warnock argument is that treating another person as a means to another's ends is "always liable to moral objection". This may be so, but what makes the moral objection valid? The original 18th century version of the moral principle, formulated by the philosopher Immanuel Kant, was that we should treat all persons (including ourselves) as ends in themselves, never as *mere* means. To be treated as ends in themselves people must be able to exercise moral agency, to make a free and informed choice to carry out acts that serve the ends of others. Payment for their services does not make people into a mere means: on the contrary lack of payment (as in slavery or breadline wages) may be much more exploitative.

4.24 Even where there is risk in an occupation (eg working as a soldier, or in the police or fire service) payment does not of itself necessarily constitute exploitation. There is unlikely to be exploitation providing that people choosing to undertake such jobs do so with full knowledge and understanding of such risks, and that the payments made to them are not of a nature or at a level to induce them to take such risks against their better judgement.

4.25 The issue of exploitation of the surrogate therefore resolves into the fundamental question of her capacity to foresee the risks entailed. Payment increases the risk of exploitation if it constitutes an inducement to participate in an activity whose degree of risk the surrogate cannot, in the nature of things, fully understand or predict. In our judgment, surrogacy does carry some unpredictable risks which become fully evident only after an agreement has been entered into, perhaps even some time after the baby has been handed over to the commissioning parents. Some women may be particularly vulnerable to these risks, because of their social, economic or personal situation. This is one of our reasons for rejecting the concept of surrogacy as a paid occupation. Even if our Terms of Reference allowed us to recommend the full commercialisation of surrogacy, we would not do so, because it would imply a normalisation of what we believe to be a difficult personal choice, with an unknown degree of psychological risk.

4.26 The degree of risk should not be exaggerated. Evidence we have received from surrogate mothers in response to our questionnaire suggests that many women have found being a surrogate an emotionally rewarding experience, with no obvious ill effects on them or their families. Others, however, describe much less happy experiences. Although there is not strong enough evidence to warrant attempts to ban surrogacy because of its effect on surrogate mothers, there is sufficient cause for concern to make regulation essential.

Welfare of the child

4.27 A second reason for restricting, or at least regulating, surrogacy is the moral imperative to make the welfare of the child our prime concern. As we have noted, we are handicapped by a lack of empirical evidence about the effect of surrogacy on the children born as the result of surrogate arrangements (or of its effect on any other children of the surrogate). Given that the risks are hard to quantify, should we give any weight to this consideration? Some writers have argued that society would have to be quite certain of substantial risks to the child before any disbenefit of being conceived in this unusual manner outweighed the benefit of life itself. After all, they argue, surely we can be confident that most disadvantaged children will still prefer life to non-existence[27].

4.28 This argument appears to us to rest on a confusion between possible and actual persons. Unless we have a belief in the pre-existence of the soul, there is no person who suffers from not being alive. A decision not to proceed with a conception because of particular circumstances - or the prevention of achieving conception because of restrictive legislation or lack of adequate resources for infertility treatment - certainly causes unhappiness and a sense of loss to the would-be *parents*. But there is no child who suffers this loss or to whom we or the parents have moral obligations.

4.29 Therefore, we do not have to show certainty of major harm to potential children before we are justified, either through personal decision or legislative restriction, in avoiding conceptions on grounds of risk to the welfare of the child. It is sufficient to show that, if such lives are brought into being, they could be significantly compromised physically or

---

27 See Harris J. *The Value of Life* Routledge, 1985, at p. 147

emotionally. By not bringing them into being we do no harm to a child, since none exists. This is not to say that people should aim for perfection in their progeny, or that the state should institute draconian measures to narrow people's procreative choices. Rather, it justifies controlling, at least to some degree, this emotionally complex way of creating a family.

4.30 In practice, welfare considerations of this kind do not lead to major incursions into procreative liberty, but to the creation of institutions which provide guidance to people with difficult procreative choices (examples of this are the provision of genetic counselling services and the HFEA guidelines within which certain fertility services are provided). In respect of surrogacy, we regard there being sufficient concern about its effects on children to justify regulation, which includes measures aimed at ensuring the best protection of the child's welfare.

Procreative liberty

4.31 However, a further objection to any restriction of this kind on procreative choice must now be considered. It has been argued[28] that the whole structure of regulation of infertility treatment recommended by Warnock and enacted in the Human Fertilisation and Embryology Act 1990 is an infringement of human rights, and constitutes discriminatory treatment of infertile people, since they are subject to restrictions not imposed upon those who can conceive by natural means. This argument gains considerable power from the much clearer evidence of likely physical or psychological damage to children in some natural conceptions[29] than any of the possible risks to children from assisted parenthood. It is outside our remit to consider the wider question of regulation of infertility treatment as a whole. However, the argument has obvious relevance to the narrower question of whether there should be any regulation of surrogacy.

4.32 We accept that people have a *prima facie* right to procreative or reproductive autonomy, and we are certainly opposed to any notion of a state-controlled licensing system[30] which prevents people from making their own procreative choices, through, for example, limits on numbers of children or enforced contraception or sterilisation. We agree that a consequence of this may be that some children are put in grave hazard by the circumstances of their conception and birth. However, we do not regard procreative autonomy as an

---

28 Harris J, correspondence submitted as evidence to the review team

29 *e.g.* women infected with the AIDS virus; drug abusers; men who are known to be potential child abusers

30 There are those, however, who do argue that all parents should be licensed by the State. See Lafollette, H "Licensing Parents", (1980) *Philosophy and Public Affairs* 1979-80 182-197

absolute right, especially since it can come into conflict with the rights of others. Procreation is not just a matter of individual freedom. It entails bringing about the life of another human, whose welfare and autonomy deserve the highest attention from the state, because of the total dependency of children on others.

4.33 In view of this, we believe that when regulation is practicable and when it does not entail major state intrusion into the lives or bodily integrity of individuals, it may be ethically justifiable. We therefore accept the appropriateness of the "welfare of the child" provision of the Human Fertilisation and Embryology Act, and believe that the principle it embodies can quite fairly be extended to surrogacy arrangements (as is presently the case in the HFEA guidelines) without an undue incursion on the rights of commissioning parents to privacy. Moreover, as we have argued earlier, the rights of the surrogate and of her children are also to be taken into account, and these must be balanced against the claims of infertile people to procreative liberty.

The gift relationship

4.34 A further ethical dimension in the surrogacy debate concerns the notion of "commodification" of childbearing entailed in surrogacy as a financial transaction. It was argued by a number of the respondents to our questionnaire that surrogacy need not be equated with "baby-selling", because any fee paid to the surrogate can be regarded as payment for the pregnancy, *ie* payment for her services, not the baby. We find it difficult to see how this distinction can be maintained, especially because any fully commercial transaction of this kind should be subject to the normal laws of contract. It is unimaginable that a commissioning couple should enter into a contract that required simply that the surrogate become pregnant and give birth. The contract would have to contain a requirement that in return for the fee the child was handed over to those contracting the pregnancy, with penalties for failure to fulfil this aspect of the agreement.

4.35 It is possible to imagine a new legislative framework, which permitted payment of a fee to the surrogate, whilst maintaining her right to retain the child, but any such legislation would rationally have to contain provision for the contracting couple to obtain redress in the event that the child was not handed over. These legal considerations lead us to the conclusion that any financial arrangement that involves remuneration rather than simply expenses[31] has to be regarded as a form of child purchase.

---

[31] The question of whether the current payment of "expenses" is really a fiction, and of what should be done about it, is dealt with in chapter 5.

4.36 We fully accept that women who offer themselves as surrogates often do so at considerable inconvenience, discomfort and risk to themselves. We have certainly no wish to encourage the exploitation of such women by creating an environment in which they are involved in such arrangements without realising that there is no financial recompense for their time and effort. But the answer to this is to make quite explicit the social values on which this activity is based. We believe that the core value here, on which many social arrangements in the United Kingdom are based, including blood and live organ donation, is the "gift relationship".

4.37 It appears that, as a society, we believe that the use of our procreative capacities to assist others should also be a gift, not a commercial transaction. (We see this value informing the policy of the HFEA to remove payment for gametes). Certainly the "cost" of the gift to the woman who undergoes pregnancy and birth in order to help an infertile couple is much greater than any other form of donation, except perhaps live kidney donation. It may be that few women will be willing to undertake such a commitment, except for a relative or close friend. But, whatever the practical consequences on the frequency of surrogacy arrangements, we have made our recommendations on the assumption that bearing a child for others should be seen within the context of a fully informed and free act of giving, and that neither the child nor the surrogate should be regarded as the subjects of a commercial transaction.

The role of law

4.38 We reject, as did the Warnock Committee, any suggestion that surrogacy arrangements should be prohibited by the criminal law. We note that other European Union states have imposed such prohibitions. In addition to the argument that no child's very existence should be subject to a "taint of criminality", we see two other objections to criminalising surrogacy *per se*. (1) Prohibition of surrogacy altogether would constitute an unjustifiable violation of the procreative liberty of the commissioning couple and the surrogate's autonomy, unless there were significant evidence that *any* form of surrogacy arrangements resulted in significant harm. We have not found such evidence. (2) Prohibition would not be effective. Unlike some other means of overcoming infertility, surrogacy is not dependent on 'high tech' medicine. Artificial insemination resulting in a partial surrogacy can and is practised without medical help or advice. Natural intercourse achieves the same end. Unless a state is prepared to police the bedrooms of the nation, surrogacy arrangements cannot effectively be outlawed, only driven underground.

4.39 We look therefore to the law to prevent effectively the commercialisation of surrogacy which we judge to be a cause of potential harm in surrogacy arrangements and to offer a system of regulation of surrogacy. In recommending regulation, albeit on a rather different model, we very much concur with the reasoning of the minority on the Warnock Committee.

4.40 The law currently seeks to restrict payments other than reasonable expenses incurred by the surrogate mother[32]. Evidence of payments made to surrogate mothers of up to £15,000 suggests that current legal rules are simply not working. For reasons outlined in Chapters 3 and 7 courts find themselves in effect "forced" to authorise expenses which are simply covert payments. There are those, among our respondents, who judge that so long as agencies do not profit from surrogacy, and so long as payments are not extortionate, this "fudge" is acceptable.

4.41 Others openly argue the case for recognising that the surrogate be paid for her labour. Women should be able to contract to offer reproductive services just as the infertility clinic is free to contract to offer IVF to establish a surrogate pregnancy. While we see the force of their argument, we believe it leads inexorably to the following consequences. (1) Payments will increase exponentially. If surrogates should be paid the economic rate for the job, payments of over £15,000 would swiftly be the norm. (2) The incidence of surrogacy would increase. The more lucrative the 'job', the more women may be attracted to it. (3) As noted earlier, if surrogacy were a commercial transaction, it should be a contract like any other and enforceable in the courts. We consider such an outcome unacceptable.

4.42 We are additionally influenced by our view that all other factors being equal, legislative policy should be consistent. The United Kingdom bans payments for organs and will soon ban payments for gametes. In both cases allowing payments would increase the supply of organs and gametes. The judgment has been made that the good to the recipient does not justify trade in bodily parts.

4.43 Nor do we judge that it can be beneficial to allow the current "fudge" to continue, even if the courts were able over time to chart a course of their own. Without intervention, payments disguised as expenses are in any case likely to rise. Undefined and unregulated, disputes about expenses add to the perils of surrogacy arrangements.

4.44 Chapter 3 described the emergence of non-profitmaking agencies willing to assist in the creation of surrogacy arrangements. We have also noted that it seems likely that other arrangements are entered into with little or no advice or guidance. Such cases are not limited to intra-family or altruistic arrangements. As did the minority in Warnock, we believe that

---

32 Otherwise obtaining a parental order or adoption may not be possible.

regulation of agencies involved in surrogacy is required. Regulation should seek both to monitor and control the activities of such organisations and, as far as possible, offer guidance on surrogacy arrangements generally. The central purpose of such regulation should be to attempt to ensure that adults do not embark on surrogacy without adequate information and advice, and that the highest priority is given to the welfare of the child to be born.

4.45 That the law should be designed to protect the welfare of children is more or less universally agreed. We acknowledge that our proposals on regulation and consequent reforms of the law seek also to protect the interests of the adults involved in surrogacy, the surrogate and the commissioning couple. Evidence as to the generally lower income and educational attainments of surrogates in comparison with that of commissioning couples, and accounts of a number of distressing experiences of surrogacy, lead us to conclude that the potential vulnerability of surrogates justifies legal protection of their welfare. Equally the passionate desire of the couple for a child and their emotional investment in the enterprise also renders them vulnerable. We believe it appropriate to seek to implement a system of regulation which (i) ensures that any third party involved in surrogacy arrangements acts appropriately and (ii) sets out guidance aimed to prevent intentional or unintentional exploitation of each other by the parties to the arrangements.

4.46 Consideration of the ethical and social dimensions of surrogacy practice in the United Kingdom in 1998, fourteen years after the Warnock Committee's initial review of surrogacy, has led us to two principal conclusions. (1) Payments for the service rendered by surrogates in bearing the child for the commissioning couple should be prohibited. Surrogates should be recompensed only for those actual expenses (including loss of earnings) occasioned by the pregnancy and the birth of the child. (2) Surrogacy arrangements should be subject to a system of regulation designed to protect the interests of all the parties involved in the arrangement. While the welfare of the child must be accorded the highest priority, evidence presented to us confirms that the nature of surrogacy arrangements are such that the adult parties, not only surrogates themselves, but commissioning couples too, are vulnerable in certain circumstances to exploitation and considerable emotional harm.

4.47 As we have noted earlier, the limited data on the progress and outcome of surrogacy arrangements make it impossible to quantify the adverse effects of surrogacy. That such effects sometimes exist, we know. We prefer to err on the side of caution in making recommendations which we hope will (i) minimise the incidence of such harm and (ii) allow surrogacy in future to be more closely monitored to ensure that data on outcomes of surrogacy arrangements become available.

Limits of the law

4.48 As chapters 5-7 will demonstrate, we do not propose to recommend that a single system of regulation be made mandatory. Parties would not be compelled to enter into surrogacy arrangements only through a licensed agency. Good practice would be set out in a Code of Practice but not enforced by the criminal courts. Parties flouting prohibitions of payments would no longer be eligible to apply for a parental order but would not be subject to criminal sanctions and may in certain circumstances still be able to adopt the child born, despite the unlawful nature of payments made.

4.49 Making mandatory resort to a regulated agency was an option most of our respondents rejected, as do we. Family arrangements, and arrangements between friends, may take place with none of the parties being aware of any new laws. In an area involving such a private sector of life we seek to use the law to ensure that those who choose to do so can obtain help with surrogacy and guidance on how to avoid its especial risks. Surrogacy will never be risk free.

4.50 Surrogacy must be approached on its very special facts. If a child is born as a result of surrogacy, however flawed ethically or socially the initial arrangement may have been, the child's welfare must be the highest priority. If the child has been entrusted to the commissioning couple, forcing the surrogate to take the child back or taking him or her into care may not promote their welfare; nor will criminalising a child's parents (including the surrogate).

4.51 In the chapters which follow we spell out in greater detail our proposals for control of payments, regulation and changes in the law, together with our reasons for these recommendations.

Chapter 5

PAYMENTS TO SURROGATES

5.1 A requirement of our terms of reference was to consider whether payments to surrogate mothers should continue to be allowed and, if so, on what basis. We were asked to examine this issue within the context that surrogacy should not be commercialised. Concern about the level of payments being made to surrogate mothers by commissioning couples was a major factor in the initiation of the present review.

The current situation

5.2 At present, surrogate mothers are entitled to receive reimbursement for genuine expenses incurred in connection with the surrogacy arrangement. No criminal offence is committed by either the surrogate mother or the commissioning couple if payments are made to the surrogate mother over and above the reimbursement of genuine expenses. In principle, such additional payments may prevent the commissioning couple from obtaining a parental order under Section 30 of the Human Fertilisation and Embryology Act 1990, or an adoption order under the terms of the Adoption Act 1976.

5.3 However, we are not aware of any case in which an application has been refused on the grounds that an unacceptably large sum of money has been paid to the surrogate mother by the commissioning couple. From the evidence that we have received during the course of the Review, it is clear that in many cases a component of the amount paid to the surrogate mother is a direct payment for services rendered rather than the reimbursement of actual expenses.

5.4 We have received accounts from COTS and elsewhere suggesting that payments of £15,000 or more are being made by commissioning couples to surrogate mothers, with a number of payments being in the range of £10,000 - £15,000.

5.5 Although systematic records of families with a child born as a result of a surrogacy arrangement have not been kept, it has been possible to obtain some information about the practice of surrogacy from Guardians *ad litem*[33].

5.6 In the 34 cases of surrogacy in which Guardians were involved, payments made to the surrogate were found to range from nothing to £12,000 (see table at Annex C). In 22%

---

33 See paragraphs 1.28-1.31

of cases where the sum paid was known, the payment was between £0 - £999 (with 16% receiving £100 or less); in 47% of cases it was between £1000 - £4999; in 28% of cases it was between £5000 - £9999; and in 3% of cases payment was more than £10,000. Payments were usually made in instalments throughout the pregnancy rather than in a lump sum.

5.7 In the light of the discrepancy between the levels of payments reported by COTS and by Guardians, it seems possible that a substantial proportion of commissioning couples are failing to apply to the courts to become the legal parents of the child. It is also possible that it is those couples who are avoiding the courts who may be paying the larger amounts to surrogate mothers.

5.8 The public consultation exercise provided information about attitudes towards payment. More than half (56%) of the respondents to the Consultation Document (excluding COTS members who generally favoured payment)[34] were against payments being made for carrying the child. However, the large majority (83%) of respondents believed that surrogate mothers should not be out of pocket as a result of their pregnancy. Those who were in favour of the payment of genuine expenses suggested that these should include, for example, maternity clothes, travel to and from the hospital to attend ante-natal clinics, and babysitting costs to allow surrogate mothers with children to attend hospital appointments.

5.9 There was less consensus in relation to loss of earnings. Seventy-five percent of respondents believed payments should include reimbursement for loss of actual earnings, but only 31% felt that surrogate mothers should be compensated for loss of potential earnings. Loss of potential earnings was considered not only to be difficult to determine but also to constitute financial benefit rather than compensation. The majority (77%) of respondents favoured the introduction of legislation to define remuneration and/or relevant expenses. Only 17% of respondents to the Consultation Document were in favour of prohibiting payment of any kind.

Problems with the current situation

5.10 From the evidence reported in paragraphs 5.4 and 5.6, it appears that payments over and above genuine expenses are being made in a substantial proportion of cases. It is also possible that aside from declared payments, additional sums are being given to surrogate mothers. A general concern raised by a number of respondents to the Consultation Document, and by some of those who gave oral evidence to the Review Team, was that

---

34 Discussion about responses to the review will be in respect of those which were identified as not being made by COTS unless otherwise stated: see paragraphs 1.37 - 1.41

payment for carrying a child commercialises the transaction.

5.11 As already discussed in Chapter 4, it is a fundamental belief in our society that children should not be viewed as commodities to be bought or sold. This principle is also enshrined in the law on adoption. Although a theoretical distinction can be made between payment for the purchase of a child and payment for a potentially risky, time-consuming and uncomfortable service, in practice it is difficult to separate the two, and it remains the case that payment other than for genuine expenses constitutes a financial benefit for the surrogate mother.

5.12 The policy of the Human Fertilisation and Embryology Authority is to withdraw payments for egg and sperm donors on the grounds that it is not appropriate for people to donate their genetic material to create new life for financial reasons. Allowing a woman to gain financially from hosting a pregnancy for someone else, whether or not her genetic material has been used, would be at odds with the spirit of gamete donation as a gift, freely and voluntarily given.

5.13 Parallels have also been drawn between surrogacy and blood or live organ donation. In the UK, bodily parts may be donated only as a gift for which no payments are allowed. We believe that surrogacy should be informed by the same values. The view that surrogacy should not take place for financial benefit is in line with the philosophy underlying the report of the Nuffield Council on Bioethics *Human Tissue: Ethical and Legal Issues* (1995), the *Council of Europe Report on Human Artificial Procreation* (1989), and Article 21 of the *Council of Europe Convention on Human Rights and Biomedicine*[35].

5.14 It is also our view that financial benefit should not influence a woman's decision to become a surrogate mother. The evidence that we have received suggests that in the absence of financial benefit many surrogate mothers would not have entered into the surrogacy arrangement. Although surrogates are also motivated by a wish to help infertile people, many are primarily motivated by payment, particularly those who have no previous connection with the commissioning couple.

5.15 Embarking on a surrogate pregnancy carries with it emotional risks in addition to the physical risks of pregnancy, and these risks may not become apparent until a pregnancy occurs. For example, the surrogate mother may regret her decision to enter into such an

---

35 *European Convention for the Protection of Human Rights and Dignity of the Human Being with regard to the Application of Biology and Medicine* (1996)

arrangement when she is expected to relinquish the baby, or later in life, perhaps when she enters into a new relationship or finds that she herself is unable to bear another child. It is worth noting in this respect that half of the surrogate mothers involved in the Guardian *ad litem* survey[36] were single at the time of the surrogate pregnancy. Given the difficulties faced by potential surrogate mothers in giving fully informed consent, we believe that the prospect of payment further complicates decision-making and results in an increased likelihood of women entering into a surrogacy arrangement when they would not otherwise have done so, particularly women experiencing financial difficulties.

5.16 Surrogacy brings with it other problems as well. The payment of a surrogate by a commissioning couple to bear a child for them creates a potentially exploitative situation, and we wish to minimise the opportunity for exploitation to occur. Although it seems that a trusting and supportive partnership can develop between the surrogate mother and the commissioning couple, the absence of payment would reduce the likelihood of undue pressure being placed on the surrogate mother.

5.17 We also wish to discourage women from becoming professional surrogates. There is evidence that some women view surrogacy as a form of employment, i.e. as an alternative to working outside the home, and a growing number of surrogates are entering into more than one surrogacy arrangement. In addition to our concerns about the physical and psychological welfare of surrogates who enter into repeated surrogacy arrangements, we also have reservations about facilitating a situation whereby some relatively poor and less educated women are having babies for their wealthier and better educated counterparts.

5.18 As discussed in Chapter 4, very little is known about the consequences for children of being born as a result of a surrogacy arrangement. Concern has been expressed regarding the potential negative effects of surrogacy for children's psychological well-being. Specifically, it has been argued that the knowledge that they had been relinquished by their surrogate mother who, in some cases, is also their genetic mother, and the knowledge that their surrogate mother had been paid to host the pregnancy, may be psychologically damaging to children. As with adopted children, failure to tell children born through surrogacy about the circumstances of their birth may place them at risk of emotional and identity problems.

5.19 The concerns regarding the potential risks to children of being born as a result of a surrogacy arrangement are purely speculative. However, in the absence of systematic data

---

[36] See annexes B and C

on what actually happens to such children, we believe, for the reasons outlined in Chapter 4, that it is not necessarily in children's best interests to learn that their surrogate mother benefitted financially from their birth or from giving them away to the commissioning couple.

5.20 In addition, we have concerns regarding the psychological consequences of surrogacy for the surrogate mother's own children. Although the Human Fertilisation and Embryology Authority Code of Practice states that in the case of surrogacy the clinic should take account of the effects of the proposed arrangement on the existing children in both families,[37] the majority of surrogacy arrangements take place outside licensed clinics.

5.21 There are also potential advantages for the commissioning couple of limiting payments to genuine expenses, in that they will not be faced with the prospect of telling a teenage child that they paid a large sum of money to the surrogate mother in order for him or her to be born. It might also be expected that surrogacy arrangements founded on altruism rather than on financial benefit would be less likely to break down. The limitation of payments would also prevent surrogate mothers from making increased financial demands on the commissioning couple once a pregnancy is established.

5.22 We appreciate that infertility can be an extremely distressing experience, and that surrogacy can provide a solution for some infertile couples. Although limiting payments to genuine expenses only is likely to reduce the number of women who wish to become surrogate mothers, we believe, for the reasons outlined above, that payments that exceed genuine expenses should not be allowed.

5.23 Whereas a surrogate mother should not gain financially from entering into a surrogacy arrangement, neither should she be expected to incur any costs as a result of a surrogate pregnancy. It is our view that women who become surrogates to help infertile couples should not suffer financial loss as a result of their altruistic act. We believe that the payment of genuine expenses does not commercialise surrogacy and thus that the payment of genuine expenses should be allowed.

Recommendations

5.24 We recommend that payments to surrogate mothers should cover only genuine expenses associated with the pregnancy. Any additional payments should be prohibited in order to prevent surrogacy arrangements being entered into for financial reasons. Details of

---

37 See paragraph 3.19b of the HFEA *Code of Practice* (July 1998)

expenses should be established before any attempt is made to create a surrogacy pregnancy, and a mechanism should be put in place to ensure that documentary evidence of expenses incurred in association with the surrogacy arrangement is produced by the surrogate mother.

5.25 We recommend that allowable expenses should be:

Maternity clothing	*Counselling fees*
Healthy food	*Legal fees*
Domestic help	*Life and disability insurance*
Travel to and from hospital/clinic	*Medical expenses*
Telephone and postal expenses	*Ovulation and pregnancy tests*
Overnight accommodation	*Insemination and IVF costs*
Child care to attend hospital/clinic	*Medicines and vitamins*

5.26 If the surrogate mother is employed when she enters into the surrogacy arrangement and has to take time off work in connection with the pregnancy or birth, her actual loss of earnings should be reimbursed. The time taken off work should be in accordance with medical advice and statutory guidelines. We would expect actual loss of earnings to be minimal, and to represent no more than the difference between the surrogate mother's usual earnings and state benefits. Documentary proof of actual loss of earnings should be provided. No compensation should be allowed for loss of potential earnings.

5.27 In the next Chapter we consider the case for regulation of surrogacy arrangements.

Chapter 6

REGULATION

6.1 We were required by our Terms of Reference to examine whether there is a case for the regulation of surrogacy arrangements through a recognised body or bodies. If we believed there was such a case, we were required to advise on the scope and operation of such arrangements.

6.2 We have extensively considered the possibility that such regulation is either unnecessary or undesirable. It might be thought, for example, that there is insufficient evidence of problems in the currently unregulated situation to justify setting up regulatory mechanisms. It has been estimated by COTS that the current "failure rate" is no more than 4%. However, we need to ask what constitutes "success" in a surrogacy arrangement. The fact that the child is handed over to the commissioning parents without contest may not be a reliable criterion of success. We have received some personal accounts of uncertainty and unhappiness among some surrogate mothers who did hand over the baby, and we remain unconvinced that all surrogacy arrangements are entered into with genuinely informed consent by all parties.

6.3 There is also uncertainty about the long-term effects of a surrogacy arrangement on the child. In the absence of reliable information on this critical issue, we believe that some form of regulation might reduce the more obvious hazards to the child and the others involved (including any children of the surrogate mother).

6.4 The situation is complicated further by the difficulty in gaining a complete and accurate picture of what is currently happening. A comparison of figures provided by Guardians *ad litem* with those provided by the Human Fertilisation and Embryology Authority, COTS and the fertility clinics suggests that there may be a considerable number of arrangements taking place outside either the informal arrangements of COTS or the procedures of the clinics. Even when COTS or other voluntary agencies have been involved, we have questions about the adequacy and impartiality of the advice and support offered to the various parties.

6.5 We have concluded, therefore, that to ensure protection of the various vulnerable parties, some form of regulation is required. But first a further objection has to be considered: even if regulation appears to be necessary, it may be undesirable because its effect would be to make the current situation worse. Some of those who are opposed to surrogacy in principle wish to avoid regulation, arguing that it will legitimise rather than discourage the practice. This was the majority view of the Warnock Report. Others, who accept surrogacy as a valid practice, fear that a stringent regulatory framework could result in driving many arrangements underground, so depriving surrogates and commissioning couples of whatever guidance is currently offered by clinics and voluntary agencies in the field.

6.6 We see some force in these arguments, particularly the latter one, but we have concluded that the risks of not having a regulatory framework are greater than any entailed by introducing one. As before, we reached this conclusion on the basis of our sense of obligation toward the several vulnerable parties in these arrangements, all of whom deserve some protection in law. We accept that it will always be possible for people to make surrogacy arrangements outside the framework of what we regard as best practice, but this possibility should not deter us from providing the best possible protection for those who do wish the benefit of a properly regulated service. The main sanction against unregulated surrogacy would be the difficulty in securing a Parental Order (see Chapter 7).

6.7 Our conclusion about the need for regulation accords with the views of the vast majority of respondents to our questionnaire, and with those of the various parties from whom we took oral evidence. Many of those opposed to surrogacy on principle still supported regulation, as did COTS and the fertility clinics currently involved in surrogacy. The differences lay in the nature of the regulatory framework proposed and in the detail of the regulations themselves, notably in relation to payment of expenses.

Options for regulation

6.8 Various options for regulatory bodies were suggested to us and others emerged during our consultations and discussions. We consider three such options below, and conclude that the most practical and effective, at least for the foreseeable future, is the third option.

Option One: Extend the Role of the Human Fertilisation and Embryology Authority (HFEA)

6.9 Many respondents favoured this option, though it should be noted that the HFEA itself did not consider it an appropriate role, at least as it is currently constituted. The regulation envisaged in this option would in effect equate surrogacy with infertility treatment, and so would require any agency providing surrogacy arrangements to be licensed by the HFEA for this purpose. At the present time 29 out of 115 licensed fertility clinics do provide surrogacy services, either through IVF or (much less commonly) artificial insemination with the commissioning father's sperm[38]. The British Fertility Society (BFS) estimates that about 60 couples a year seek IVF surrogacy from these clinics and this represents only 0.2% of all IVF cycles annually.

6.10 Since this option envisages an extension of the HFEA's role to provide oversight of all surrogacy arrangements, there are only two ways in which this could be achieved. The first would be to require that all authorised surrogacy had to take place in a licensed fertility clinic. This is the mechanism favoured by the BFS, who argued in their submission to us that regulation should make it "necessary for all surrogacy arrangements, IVF and natural, to go through a proper process of medical assessment, counselling and review by an Ethics Committee." This, the BFS claimed, would be best achieved by bringing all arrangements under the care of HFEA licensed fertility clinics, preferably in a limited number of specialist regional centres.

6.11 The alternative possibility is that surrogacy could continue both in clinics but also through "natural methods", under the auspices of non-medical bodies like COTS. The HFEA would be required to licence *both* types of agency.

6.12 An obvious advantage of the first form of this option is that by restricting all surrogacy to fertility clinics the risk of transmission of infection to the surrogate and the child would be avoided. Self-insemination carries with it some risk of infection such as HIV and hepatitis, not all of which can be excluded by prior testing of the commissioning father. There are documented cases of the transmission of HIV through artificial insemination, despite prior testing. This is because of the latency period before HIV infection is detectable. This risk would be avoided in licensed fertility clinics, since they use only cryo-preserved sperm, with the donor being retested after a six month waiting period.

6.13 However, we have rejected this option, for a number of reasons. Although infertility is clearly a reason for seeking surrogacy, we do not believe that surrogacy arrangements are correctly perceived as merely another treatment for infertile people. The involvement of the surrogate mother requires a consideration of other factors, much more akin to the dilemmas of adoption than those of infertility, both from the point of view of her welfare and of the child's welfare. We do not believe, therefore, that fertility clinics are necessarily the correct setting for negotiating surrogacy arrangements, though we accept that they have an important part to play, especially in IVF surrogacy.

---

38 See paragraph 1.23

6.14 We have noted that clinics currently offering IVF surrogacy are not and cannot currently become involved in those aspects of the arrangement which are our main concern: the circumstances of the commissioning parents, the selection of surrogates, and the nature of the agreement between the parties. We repeat the point that surrogacy should not be viewed as just another treatment option for infertility.

6.15 It should be noted that on the evidence available to us, it appears that at least two thirds of all conceptions arising from surrogacy arrangements take place outside licensed fertility clinics. Of the third or so conducted under the auspices of licensed clinics most are IVF surrogacies. Only 9% of the pregnancies involving medical oversight reported in the Guardians *ad litem* survey (see Annex C) resulted from medically supervised insemination. Should surrogacy be limited to treatment in licensed clinics, surrogacy may come to be perceived as simply another treatment option. Criteria governing the provision of treatment may be expanded to allow increasingly for surrogacy to be offered as an alternative to failed IVF, perhaps at an even earlier stage in treatment. The cost of attempts at IVF re-enforced by a requirement to pay clinic fees for surrogacy could act as an incentive to make surrogacy, sooner rather than later, an attractive option.

6.16 Additionally at present couples resorting to surrogacy do not appear, in the majority of cases, to seek licensed treatment, opting instead for partial surrogacy on a more informal basis. We recognise the dangers of "do-it-yourself" surrogacy. However, since there is no general prohibition on self-insemination with fresh sperm, it is difficult to see how a special prohibition operating only in relation to surrogate pregnancies could or should be enforced.

6.17 We therefore consider that the case for requiring that surrogacy arrangements take place only in licensed fertility clinics is not a strong one. The problem of transmission of infection in self-insemination is serious, but we suggest (in later paragraphs of this chapter) that recommendations for safe insemination be included in a Code of Practice for all agencies arranging surrogacy. A woman opting for self-insemination would then be able to do so with fully informed consent, with a clear understanding of the risks.

6.18 For similar reasons to the above, we do not favour the alternative version of this option, which would extend the role of the HFEA to include oversight and licensing of all agencies involved in surrogacy, whether or not they were fertility clinics. We do not regard this as an appropriate role for the Authority. We are supported in this view by the submission of the HFEA itself, which states its position as follows:

The HFEA regulates the medical treatments required by the surrogate mother in order to become pregnant in a surrogacy arrangement. The nature of the regulation required for surrogacy agencies is outside the HFEA's remit and area of expertise...

...the role of surrogacy agencies is to match up surrogate mothers with commissioning couples and to support the surrogacy arrangement after pregnancy has been achieved which can include the subsequent registration of birth, adoption or the obtaining of a parental order for the child. The body regulating surrogacy agencies would need to have knowledge and expertise in those areas, and not the medical and scientific expertise covered by the HFEA.

6.19 We agree with the HFEA about the different expertise required, but in addition we think that any attempt to extend the remit of the HFEA (for example, by setting up a special subcommittee with the range of expertise required) would fail to reflect the unique nature of surrogacy arrangements. The context within which the HFEA operates is essentially a medical one, but for the surrogate mother and the child she carries and gives birth to, the main issues are psychological, social and legal. Medical issues do arise in IVF surrogacy, but these are already fully regulated by the HFEA. We are concerned with the wider issues which lie outside the medical context.

Option Two: A New Licensing Authority

6.20 A second option would be to set up a licensing authority specifically for the oversight and control of surrogacy. Such a body (which might be called the Surrogacy Licensing Authority) could have a range of functions, including the licensing and inspection of agencies involved in surrogacy arrangements, the drawing up of a Code of Practice or of regulations governing the practice of surrogacy, the compilation of statistics on surrogacy, the promotion of research into its outcomes, and advice to Government on future legislation or regulation in light of new developments. The Authority would be composed of people with a range of knowledge and experience, including both providers and recipients of services related to surrogacy, and it would require appropriate administrative support. Consideration would have to be given as to how it would be funded, *e.g.* by a levy on surrogacy agencies or by central government funding from an appropriate government department.

6.21 This option has some obvious advantages. It would provide comprehensive expert advice to all those involved in surrogacy and would clearly separate surrogacy from infertility services. By means of the Code of Practice and the licensing procedures, it would ensure that arrangements were made in a professional manner, including effective methods for selection and screening of commissioning parents and surrogate mothers, and that appropriate counselling and continuing support was offered to all involved parties, without bias toward either commissioning couples or surrogates. It would provide the Courts with a set of criteria by which to judge the appropriateness of granting or withholding Parental Orders to commissioning couples. And, last but by no means least, it would ensure more accurate records of the volume and nature of surrogacy arrangements in the United Kingdom, providing the basis for future research into its long-term effects on the parties involved, particularly the children.

6.22 We have, however, decided to reject this option on the ground that it would entail creating a complex and expensive regulatory arrangement, in a situation whose future development is by no means clear. This point will be particularly cogent if our recommendations on the regulation of expenses paid to surrogate mothers are accepted (see chapter 5 above). We do not envisage any increase in the number of surrogacy arrangements, if there is no financial advantage to women in becoming surrogate mothers - indeed there may well be a sharp decrease. We estimate that currently there are between 100 to 180 surrogacy arrangements[39] and perhaps 50 to 80 surrogacy births[40] in England each year.[41] This is very different from the annual volume of infertility treatments and the number of fertility clinics in both the public and private sector, which clearly require a licensing authority like the HFEA. In light of this, the creation of a "Surrogacy Licensing Authority" could be seen as an excessive reaction to current concerns about the practice of surrogacy. Moreover, we believe that most, if not all, of the advantages of setting up a new authority can be achieved by our third, much simpler, option.

---

39 For example, the British Fertility Society estimates that there are about 60 couples requiring treatment by IVF surrogacy each year. If this represents nearly one-third of all surrogacy arrangements (see paragraph 6.15) then the total number of arrangements will be (60+120) = 180

40 For example, if we use the figures provided by Guardians *ad litem* for our survey in England (see paragraph 1.31), 21% of the surrogacy births in which they were involved followed IVF treatment in clinics licensed by the HFEA and 79% used self-insemination (or, in a very small number of cases, medically assisted insemination). We know that there were 10 IVF surrogacy births in 1995 (the last full year for which figures are available). If these represent about 21% of all surrogacy births then the number of 'self-insemination' births will be about 38; and the total will be (38+10) = 48

41 We have no doubt that, were surrogacy put on a commercial footing, as some of our respondents advocated, and there were a financial benefit to being a surrogate, there would be a substantially greater number. Evidence from the USA shows that commercial surrogacy can be a very successful business venture.

Third Option: Registration by the UK Health Departments

6.23 In this third option all agencies involved in surrogacy arrangements would be required to be registered by the UK Health Departments and to operate in accordance with a statutory Code of Practice, but no new Authority would be set up. As a first step the Department of Health, in consultation with the other UK Health Departments, would draw up a Code of Practice after discussion with relevant bodies and individuals. We believe that this option has the merit of simplicity and that the Health Departments already have relevant experience of registration procedures of this kind.[42]

6.24 Clearly some additional resource would be required, but this would be much less than that entailed in creating and supporting a new authority. As an interim measure (prior to the necessary legislation) the Departments would draw up and promulgate a voluntary code and invite relevant bodies to seek voluntary registration. The Code would also be drawn to the attention of professional bodies and of the HFEA, so that they could consider incorporating relevant aspects of it into the guidance they issue to practitioners and clinics.

6.25 Although the Code will of necessity be modified and refined during the consultation process and with experience of its use during the interim period, we consider that it must contain the following broad provisions[43]:

- a statement of allowable expenses, as defined in paragraph 5.25 - 5.26 above;

- a description of the range of information which must be made available to all parties prior to any agreement being reached, including clear guidance on the legal aspects and a guarantee of access to independent legal advice (at no expense to the surrogate);

- procedures for the minimisation of physical risk to the surrogate and the child (*e.g.* safe insemination methods);

- criteria for minimum counselling and follow-up procedures to be made available to all parties;

- criteria for the selection of both commissioning couples and surrogates; and

---

42 *eg* in respect of the approval of private sector abortion clinics and registration of Pregnancy Advice Bureaux

43 See Chapter 8 for additional guidance *re* Code of Practice.

- a model memorandum of understanding between the parties.

6.26 In addition to the Code, the Health Departments would also need to give consideration to establishing requirements for full record keeping; reporting of specified statistics; and clear guidelines on how research will be facilitated into the outcomes of the arrangements, with a description of appropriate procedures for independent ethical appraisal of all proposed research projects.

Chapter 7

REFORMING THE LAW

Introduction

7.1 Our Terms of Reference required us to consider whether, in the light of our findings and recommendations in relation to the continuation of payments to surrogate mothers and regulation of surrogacy arrangements, changes were needed to the Surrogacy Arrangements Act 1985 and/or section 30 of the Human Fertilisation and Embryology Act 1990. It will be apparent from the preceding two chapters of our Report that we have concluded that such changes are necessary and that legislative reform is required to ensure that surrogacy arrangements in the United Kingdom are adequately regulated and monitored.

7.2 We recommend that consideration be given to the repeal of both the Surrogacy Arrangements Act 1985 and section 30 of the Human Fertilisation and Embryology Act 1990, and their replacement by a new Surrogacy Act. The Surrogacy Act would seek to address in the one statute the main legal principles governing surrogacy arrangements in the United Kingdom, to offer a surrogacy "code".

7.3 Very briefly, we envisage that the Surrogacy Act would:

(i) provide for the continuation of the current provisions of Section 1A of the 1985 Act relating to the non-enforceability of surrogacy contracts;

(ii) provide for the continuation of current provisions prohibiting commercial agencies from assisting in the creation of surrogacy arrangements and related provisions prohibiting advertisements in relation to surrogacy arrangements;

(iii) introduce new statutory provisions defining and limiting lawful payments to surrogate mothers;

(iv) provide for the promulgation by the UK Health Departments of a Code of Practice governing surrogacy arrangements generally;

(v) provide for the registration of non profit-making surrogacy agencies by the Health Departments and that such agencies will be required to comply with the Departments' Code of Practice on surrogacy arrangements;

(vi) prohibit the operation of unregistered agencies;

(vii) establish new provisions for the grant of a parental order to commissioning couples (a revised section 30 order);

(viii) provide that parental orders shall be made only where the parties concerned have complied with the provisions of the Surrogacy Act.

7.4 In addition to our recommendations for the enactment of a new Surrogacy Act, we also recommend certain interim measures to control surrogacy practice at a voluntary level prior to legislation coming into force, and certain other measures requiring amendment of secondary legislation only, which we believe can, and should, be implemented immediately.

7.5 We also recommend that the Department of Health invites relevant professional bodies, such as the General Medical Council (GMC), the United Kingdom Central Council for Nursing, Midwifery and Health Visiting (UKCC), the Royal College of Nursing, the Royal College of Midwives and the Medical Royal Colleges, to take notice of our Report and consider whether, and, if so how, the Surrogacy Act's Code of Practice should be addressed in their own professional ethical guidelines.

A New Surrogacy Act

7.6 We thought long and hard before recommending the introduction of a new Surrogacy Act. We remain aware of the paucity of evidence on the practice of surrogacy and its long term consequences for all those involved. Ensuring such evidence can be obtained and evaluated so that legal provisions controlling surrogacy meet the real needs of the individuals concerned and the legitimate interests of society is crucial. We explored the options for recommending entirely voluntary additional regulation of surrogacy arrangements, in particular of payments made to surrogate mothers, and of organisations involved in assisting in such arrangements.

7.7 We concluded however that it was unlikely that such a voluntary scheme (implemented without any prospect of timely legislation) would operate to reverse what we perceive to be a trend leading, if not to increased "commercialisation" of surrogacy, at least to its "professionalisation", a trend which we have already described as undesirable and fraught with risks to those involved. In the absence of a significant incentive to comply with measures to control organisations involved with surrogacy arrangements, we doubted that such organisations would do so. This was because, in particular, some of our recommendations, particularly with regard to payments, go against the deeply held and very genuine opinions of some of those organisations (notably COTS).

7.8 Moreover, limiting payments as we recommend seemed equally unlikely to be attainable without (at least ultimately) statutory definition of permissible payments and the introduction of sanctions to enforce such limitations primarily by means of a revised procedure for parental orders. We also concluded that it was only with statutory powers that the Health Departments were likely to be able to monitor and obtain the evidence of surrogacy practice which we believe to be essential.

7.9 As we explain in Chapter 4 of our Report we reject the views expressed by a number of consultees that surrogacy be regarded as just another variant of assisted conception. We consider surrogacy to be a practice involving social and ethical dimensions of a different kind and order to other forms of assisted conception. The arrangement inherent in both "partial" and "full" surrogacy which requires a woman to bear a child to be entrusted to the care of others, albeit at least one of those others may be the child's genetic parent, creates a set of circumstances more closely analogous to adoption than other forms of fertility treatment. The especial vulnerability of all those involved in surrogacy must not be underestimated. We consider that legislative arrangements in relation to surrogacy are thus best provided in a single Act of Parliament recognising the special nature of surrogacy and seeking to make comprehensive provision for its regulation.

7.10 Our terms of reference excluded any consideration of reversing fundamental principles (embodied in the 1985 Act) prohibiting the operation of commercial agencies (as in some parts of the USA) and ensuring that a surrogate mother could not be compelled to give up her child i.e. that surrogacy contracts remain unenforceable. However, as we explained above, our conclusions on the practice of surrogacy positively supports both the current ban on commercial agencies and the non-enforceability of surrogacy contracts. Any new Surrogacy Act should thus consolidate most of the provisions of the 1985 Act. We now address new provisions to be included in the proposed Surrogacy Act.

Payments

7.11 We propose that our recommendations in relation to limiting payments to the actual and provable expenses occasioned to the surrogate mother be given statutory force. The Surrogacy Act should provide for a broad definition of lawful expenses but one that goes beyond the current laconic reference in section 30 of the 1990 Act to "expenses reasonably incurred". The statutory definition should expressly exclude potential loss of earnings, and provide authority to ensure expenses can be proven. Provisions in the Act defining expenses in broad terms of principle should also empower Ministers to issue directions on what constitutes reasonable expenses and the methods by which expenses shall be proven.

7.12 As failure to comply with the statutory limitations on payments would under our proposals result in ineligibility for a parental order, regulations made under the Surrogacy Act relating to the grant of such orders and in particular the powers and duties of Guardians *ad litem* must ensure that Guardians are empowered to require adequate evidence of all payments claimed to constitute expenses.

7.13 We have given careful consideration to whether if our proposed limitations on payments is to be effective (as current provisions are not), sanctions other than ineligibility for a parental order should be imposed. Such sanctions could take two forms.

(i) More draconian "penalties" could be imposed on commissioning couples in relation to their ability to establish themselves as the child's legal parents, for example, by making them ineligible to adopt the child. We ruled out such options because of the adverse impact on the welfare of the child. In the majority of cases where unlawful payments may have been made, the child will nonetheless be in the care of the commissioning couple and the surrogate mother will not desire his or her return. Refusal of a parental order indicates society's disapproval of payments made and puts the couple to the added burden of seeking adoption. The adoption process allows separate legal representation for the child and ensures a full examination of the couple's suitability to parent the child. The adoption judge can ultimately review the level of any payments made and decide whether to exercise his powers in all the circumstances to give retrospective authorisation to such payments. The adoption court enjoys the necessary powers to give full weight to the welfare of the child. Prohibiting an application for adoption, where unlawful payments may have been made would risk commissioning couples, even more regularly than now, seeking to avoid any formal steps to acquire joint parental responsibilities in respect of the child. Children would be living with a couple where the "social" mother had no legal relationship with the child and the surrogate retains parental responsibility. Such a state of affairs risks disrupting the security of the child should the adults involved in his or her creation later come into dispute.

(ii) The commissioning couple and/or the surrogate mother could be fined an amount representing the excess of the payment over permissible expenses. The adoption court could be granted such a power to fine the applicants or a separate criminal offence created. Criminalising payments to the surrogate, however, remains open to two objections. (1) Does that criminalisation, as Warnock held, subject the very birth of the child to a taint of criminality? (2) Will the invocation of the criminal law drive couples to avoid any formal, legal process to acquire parental status in relation to the child? We conclude that the potential harm to the child involved in criminalising the couple or the surrogate outweighs any argument that effective sanctions to limit payments must include in the last resort the use of the criminal process.

7.14 Our rejection of sanctions, additional to ineligibility for a parental order, to enforce prohibitions of payments will have to be considered carefully in the light of proposals from the Lord Chancellor's Department on July 2 1998 that unmarried fathers who register the birth jointly with their child's mother should automatically acquire parental responsibility in relation to that child. Such proposals have significant implications for our recommendations.

7.15 If these proposals are enacted the genetic father in a surrogacy arrangement may, in some circumstances, acquire parental responsibility by registering the child jointly with the surrogate. This creates a risk that where prohibition of payments has been violated and/or other requirements of the Code of Practice have not been complied with the child will simply be entrusted to his or her legal father, and no application for either a parental or adoption order will be made. The child will have no legal relationship with his or her commissioning mother and the surrogate will retain parental responsibility in relation to a child with whom she may have no regular contact. Should the commissioning couple's relationship break down, or disputes later arise between the surrogate and either or both partners of the commissioning couple, the potential exists for harmful conflict damaging to the child. Additionally the commissioning mother could find herself at a substantial disadvantage in any dispute about the child's future.

A Code of Practice

7.16 The Surrogacy Act would make provision for the appropriate UK Health Departments (in consultation with the Human Fertilisation and Embryology Authority) to promulgate a Code of Practice relating to surrogacy arrangements. That Code of Practice should embody the key principles of good practice outlined above. We offer some further guidance on the content of such a Code in Chapter 8.

7.17 The Code of Practice would be binding on registered agencies. Compliance with the Code would be a condition of registration and breach of the Code grounds for deregistration.

7.18 However, we also propose that the Code of Practice should operate as an *advisory* Code to provide guidance in relation to all surrogacy arrangements whether made through a registered agency or privately. Provisions of the Code of Practice designed to protect the interests of all parties and to ensure that those who embark on surrogacy arrangements do so on the basis of sufficient information and adequate counselling would be applicable to any form of arrangement, be the arrangement recompensed by expenses, or entirely altruistic. Those who elect not to use a registered agency to assist in the creation of a surrogacy arrangement could, nonetheless, look to the Code as a statement of good practice. To seek to ensure that the provisions of the Code are made known to parties entering into purely altruistic and/or intra-familial arrangements, we make recommendations below to ensure that all professionals likely to be involved in surrogacy and Guardians *ad litem* are fully conversant with the provisions of the Code.

7.19 Our Terms of Reference focused on issues of payment and regulation in relation to surrogacy arrangements. We have rejected proposals to allow overt payment for surrogacy services. It should not however be assumed that we regard altruistic surrogacy as unproblematic. Where a sister, cousin or close friend is unable to bear a child, the pressure on a potential surrogate to assist her may be extreme. Measures to attempt to ensure that any consent given to act as a surrogate is free and informed are as crucial in altruistic as in other forms of surrogacy. Concern about the welfare of the child, the surrogate and the commissioning couple should be just as important. Where an aunt is also in some sense the mother of a child there is potential for family conflict harmful to all those involved. The psychological risk to the surrogate of bearing and handing over a child even to a beloved sister is just as great. Accordingly we would want to see the Code of Practice addressing fully the need for guidance in altruistic surrogacy, and to encourage parties contemplating such an arrangement to seek assistance from a registered surrogacy agency.

7.20 As we propose above, the Code of Practice would be promulgated by the UK Departments of Health in consultation with the HFEA. We recommend that such parts of the Code of Practice of surrogacy which are relevant to the operation of licensed clinics might additionally be considered by the HFEA for incorporation into their own Code of Practice and so be binding on licensed clinics. This might include provisions as to minimum age of surrogates, gaps between pregnancies and maximum number of surrogate pregnancies. The HFEA should be invited to consider requiring licensed clinics to take reasonable steps to ensure that any couple presenting with a potential surrogate had understood and complied with provisions relating to payments, use of registered agencies, and the need for counselling.

Registration of agencies

7.21 The Surrogacy Act would provide for registration by the Department of Health of non-profitmaking organisations who are engaged in the introduction of commissioning couples to potential surrogate mothers. Registration would be conditional on establishing that an organisation has sufficient expertise to operate in relation to surrogacy arrangements and agrees to comply with the Code of Practice. Registered agencies would be obliged to furnish details of all surrogacy arrangements to the Department. The Act would make it a criminal offence for any organisation or individual to assist in the creation of a surrogacy arrangement, unless such an organisation (or individual) is registered with the Department of Health pursuant to the Surrogacy Act.

Revised parental order

7.22 A commissioning couple would be eligible to apply for a parental order *only* if they can establish that they have complied with the statutory limitations on payments. The revised order would *not* authorise the judge to approve otherwise impermissible payments. The revised order would further provide that applicants for a parental order should additionally establish compliance with the Code of Practice. For example, use of an unregistered agency would be in breach of the Code of Practice. However, save in relation to payments, the judge before whom the application for the order is made should be empowered to excuse inadvertent non-compliance where all the circumstances suggested that the arrangement had been concluded in good faith.

7.23 If, however, neither the couple nor the surrogate were aware of the requirement that agencies be registered, their lack of knowledge would not preclude the grant of a parental order where all the other conditions for granting such an order were met. (The agency would still be liable for prosecution for operating without registration). By contrast, were it to be established that to the knowledge of the commissioning couple the surrogate was only 16 and no attempt had been made to provide her with adequate advice or counselling, the judge might well be disinclined to exercise his or her discretion to grant a parental order.

7.24 In addition to the current conditions embodied in section 30 of the 1990 Act, we recommend that the following additional provisions should be made either in the Act or regulations made under it (or other appropriate legislation) in order to ensure that the welfare of the child is better protected:

- <u>Parental orders should be obtained only in the High Court</u>

  The particular and complex issues inherent in surrogacy arrangements are such that we suggest that all applications for parental orders should be heard in the Family Division of the High Court. Such a measure would ensure that the effective "approval" of a surrogacy arrangement is given by judges of the highest experience. The child's interests would be represented by the Guardian *ad litem*, who could have separate legal representation. Centralising applications for parental orders would also result in the development of the necessary expertise by a small group of judges and would allow similarly for a small panel of Guardians to specialise in surrogacy. Current arrangements whereby magistrates may be confronted at random with one or two applications for parental orders are unsatisfactory.

- Judges should be able to order DNA tests

In order for a parental order to be granted in accordance with section 30 of the 1990 Act, surrogacy arrangements must involve a *pre-conceptual* agreement whereby a woman undertakes to bear a child who is genetically related to at least one of the commissioning couple. It has been suggested to us that on occasion Guardians have had doubts about whether any such genetic relationship to the child exists. Judges should be empowered to require DNA tests to establish such a relationship. Without such powers, the possibility arises that women who are already pregnant may be persuaded to agree to give up the child at birth under cover of an assumed surrogacy arrangement. We have also been told of cases of pre-conceptual arrangements where a surrogate agrees to carry a child unrelated to either of the commissioning couple *ie* an embryo created by donor gametes. In such a case there would currently be no eligibility for a parental order nor do we judge that there should be. These cases amount in effect to pre-natal adoption agreements and should be governed by the general laws relating to adoption. Surrogacy must not become a device by which to evade adoption laws.

- Guardians *ad litem* should have powers to check criminal records

Guardians expressed great concern to us about their present lack of power to check criminal records to ascertain whether the commissioning couple have any criminal convictions likely to endanger the welfare of the child. While we judge that only rarely will couples prove to have such convictions, when the law is invoked to entrust a child to the commissioning parents, and to sever any links with the surrogate who gave birth to him or her, it is a fundamental pre-requisite of protection of the child's welfare to ensure that his or her prospective parents have no record of child abuse or related criminal conduct.

- The commissioning couple should be habitually resident in the United Kingdom, the Channel Islands or the Isle of Man for a period of 12 months immediately preceding the application for a parental order.

  Section 30 as presently drafted requires that the couple or at least one of them be domiciled in the United Kingdom, the Channel Islands or the Isle of Man. Common law domicile has become a concept of tortuous complexity and it is possible to be domiciled in a country with which the person has at best only tenuous links. We therefore recommend that section 30 be amended to provide for the more straightforward test of habitual residence. It is our view that the condition of habitual residence should apply to both members of the commissioning couple.

Professional ethical guidelines

7.25 Our recommendations seek to ensure that couples who resort to surrogacy are able to do so on an informed basis and in a manner that minimises the potential dangers of such arrangements. Couples who elect to use an agency should be able to rely on the expertise of that agency and to pursue their arrangement through an approved Code of Practice. We do not however propose that use of a registered agency be made mandatory. We recognise that private arrangements will continue and that at least initially some couples resorting to surrogacy will be entirely unaware of the legislative framework within which we propose surrogacy arrangements should be regulated.

7.26 We therefore recommend that the UK Departments of Health consult with all the professional bodies whose members may be in professional contact with individuals contemplating involvement in surrogacy. We propose that the Departments bring this Report to the attention of the relevant regulatory bodies, including the General Medical Council, the United Kingdom Central Council for Nursing, Midwifery and Health Visiting, and the Law Society, and invite them to take steps to ensure that practitioners are aware of principles embodied in the Surrogacy Act and the Code of Practice. The Royal College of Obstetricians and Gynaecologists, the Royal College of General Practitioners, the Royal College of Nursing and the Royal College of Midwives (whose members are most likely to be in regular contact with patients involved in surrogacy arrangements) should be asked to consider incorporating relevant provisions of the Code of Practice in their own ethical guidance to members. A similar approach should be made to, among others, the British Association of Social Workers, the British Infertility Counsellors Association, the British Association of Counselling and the British Psychological Society.

7.27 We recommend that the professions are encouraged to take steps to ensure that members both comply with the Code of Practice insofar as it relates to their own practice and take reasonable steps to bring the Code of Practice to the attention of patients and clients. The regulatory bodies of the relevant professions should be invited to consider whether providing professional assistance in the operation of unregistered surrogate agencies should be designated as professional misconduct.

7.28 To assist further in the dissemination of the Code of Practice, active steps should be taken to bring this Report and the Code to the attention of other interested bodies, such as the British Medical Association, and to publicise the Code to the public at large.

Immediate action

7.29 We recommend that existing secondary legislation be amended so that parental orders can be obtained only in the High Court.

Interim measures

7.30 We recommend that consultation between the Health Departments, the HFEA and other interested parties as to a draft Code of Practice begin as soon as possible. Once any necessary administrative mechanisms are in place, the Departments should invite organisations currently involved, or who might wish to be involved, in surrogacy arrangements to apply for voluntary registration.

Chapter 8

A NOTE ON A DRAFT CODE OF PRACTICE

8.1 The promulgation of a Code of Practice defining minimum standards of good practice in relation to surrogacy arrangements is central to our recommendations in Chapters 6 and 7 for the regulation of surrogacy. The Code of Practice will need to be developed in consultation with all the bodies currently involved in the practice of surrogacy and is likely to draw on guidelines already developed by bodies such as the BMA. The Code will be binding on registered agencies and act as a model of good practice to guide all those contemplating entering into a surrogacy arrangement.

8.2 The detailed content of such a Code of Practice will be for the Department of Health to settle after the necessary consultation process. On the basis of the evidence presented to us, we offer the following recommendations in relation to the key elements of any Code of Practice governing surrogacy arrangements.

8.3 The Code must clearly spell out the basis on which surrogacy arrangements are permissible in the United Kingdom. It should state unequivocally that surrogacy arrangements are unenforceable in the courts, that only defined levels of allowable expenses may be paid to the surrogate, and that the welfare of the child must be the paramount concern of all parties to the arrangement, the courts and all other agencies involved. The risks of surrogacy to all involved in such arrangements must be spelled out.

8.4 In relation to the child, the Code must as a minimum address the following issues. It must be established that both the surrogate and the commissioning couple have given the requisite consideration to the child's welfare. The commissioning couple must be able to demonstrate that they are able to care for the child and have adequately considered questions of continuing contact between the surrogate and the child and whether, how and when the child will be informed of the circumstances of his or her birth. At present no-one under 18 can apply for a parental order. Consideration must be given to a higher minimum age for commissioning parents and to a maximum age. Where a couple resort to surrogacy because the intending mother suffers from a medical condition making pregnancy dangerous to her, there must be clear evidence that nonetheless she is able to rear the child.

8.5 In relation to other children of the surrogate or the commissioning couple, it should be established that the impact on them of the birth of the child born as a result of the surrogacy arrangement has been fully considered.

8.6 In relation to the surrogate, the Code must as a minimum ensure the following. The surrogate must be provided with comprehensive information about the risks, physical and psychological, entailed in surrogate pregnancy and relinquishing a child. She should have access to independent counselling and legal advice. A period of reflection between any initial approach to act as a surrogate and any attempt to establish a pregnancy should be prescribed. Clear information should be provided on the possible means of establishing pregnancy and the potential risks of unsupervised self insemination should be spelled out. Where a surrogate is proposing to bear a child for a friend or relative the importance of free, informed consent in such altruistic arrangements and the risks particular to such arrangements should be detailed.

8.7 In order to safeguard better the welfare and interests of surrogates, the following additional issues should be addressed in the Code. There should be a minimum age (we propose 21) to act as a surrogate (we received an account of a minor being approached to undertake a surrogate pregnancy). There should also be a maximum age. Adequate procedures to screen the surrogate's health and minimise the physical risks of pregnancy must be in place.

8.8 The surrogate should have given birth and have living with her at least one child of her own. A minimum period (we recommend two years) should elapse between any pregnancies. We received accounts of surrogates being persuaded to embark on a second pregnancy within weeks of giving birth. In line with our opinion that surrogacy should not be seen as a profession, a maximum number of occasions on which a woman acts as a surrogate should be laid down. We recommend that the norm be on one occasion only, save where a commissioning couple seek a sibling for a previous child where the surrogate was the genetic mother.

8.9 In relation to commissioning couples, the Code should as a minimum address the following. The risks of surrogacy arrangements must be spelled out as should the legal consequences for both partners. The importance of taking steps to secure their legal relationship with the child by means of an application for a parental order or adoption should be addressed. Commissioning couples should be required to undertake whatever legal steps are necessary to ensure the child's security. Surrogacy should remain an option of the last resort available only to couples where the intending mother's condition renders pregnancy impossible or highly dangerous to her. What constitutes impossibility and whether repeated failed IVF cycles are a sufficient ground to resort to surrogacy should be clarified.

8.10 To minimise the legal risks attaching to surrogacy arrangements both partners should be habitually resident in the United Kingdom, the Channel Islands or the Isle of Man.

8.11 In relation to professionals involved in surrogacy, the Code should define minimum standards, especially for counselling.

8.12 The Code should stress the value in all surrogacy arrangements (including intra-familial and other altruistic arrangements) of drawing up a memorandum of understanding, defining and clarifying the expectations of the parties. That memorandum should record the parties' arrangements to secure the future welfare of the child, including agreements about contact between the surrogate and the child and/or what the child is to be told about his or her origins. It should address how pregnancy is to be established and what screening processes pre-conceptually and pre-natally are agreed to safeguard the health of the surrogate and the child.

8.13 Issues relating to the conduct of pregnancy should be addressed, such as any undertaking the surrogate may have offered in relation to smoking, alcohol, diet and ante-natal care. Arrangements for the commissioning couple to keep in contact with and provide support for the surrogate in the course of pregnancy must be spelled out. What arrangements will follow the birth for the child to be entrusted to the couple, and how the couple will acquire joint parental responsibility in relation to the child should be agreed. What is to happen in certain contingencies such as the detection of fetal abnormality, miscarriage, stillbirth, the birth of a disabled child, or injury to or the death of the surrogate herself should be agreed. Arrangements for the provision of life and disability cover for the surrogate should be included.

8.14 The Code must emphasise the non-contractual nature of any memorandum of understanding while explaining the importance of all parties setting out as clearly as possible their expectations of each other. It may be that when the Code of Practice is drafted a model memorandum of understanding could be appended to it.

8.15 In addition, the Department(s) will need to establish specifications for agencies which are eligible for licensing including: professional standards to be met; methods of funding (commercial agencies will remain illegal); accountability; constitution and procedures; and record keeping (including the length of time for retention) and the requirements for statistical reporting to the Department(s).

8.16 Guidelines will also need to be established for the facilitation of research through adequate record keeping, procedures for full consent to research and methods of independent ethical appraisal.

Chapter 9

SUMMARY OF RECOMMENDATIONS

We recommend:

Payments

1. Payments to surrogate mothers should cover only genuine expenses associated with the pregnancy (paragraph 5.24).

2. Additional payments should be prohibited in order to prevent surrogacy arrangements being entered into for financial benefit (paragraph 5.24).

3. The basis on which expenses will be met should be established before any attempt is made to create a surrogacy pregnancy, with a requirement for documentary evidence of expenses incurred in association with the surrogacy arrangement to be produced by the surrogate mother (paragraph 5.24).

4. Legislation should define expenses in broad terms of principle and empower Ministers to issue directions on what constitutes reasonable expenses and the methods by which expenses shall be proven (paragraph 7.11).

Regulation

5. Agencies involved in surrogacy arrangements should be required to be registered by the UK Health Departments and to operate in accordance with the Code of Practice required under the terms of the proposed new Surrogacy Act (paragraph 6.23).

6. The Department of Health, in consultation with the other UK Health Departments, should draw up a Code of Practice after discussion with relevant bodies and individuals. The Code should be binding on registered agencies. The Code should also operate as an *advisory* Code to provide guidance in relation to all surrogacy arrangements whether made through a registered agency or privately (paragraph 6.23).

7. As an interim measure (prior to the necessary legislation) the UK Health Departments should draw up and promulgate a voluntary code and invite relevant bodies to seek voluntary registration. The Code should also be drawn to the attention of professional bodies and of the Human Fertilisation and Embryology Authority, so that they could consider incorporating advice on relevant aspects of it into the guidance they issue to practitioners and clinics

(paragraph 6.24).

8. In addition to the Code, the Health Departments should also consider establishing requirements for full record keeping and reporting of specified statistics; and clear guidelines on how research will be facilitated into the outcomes of the arrangements (paragraph 6.26).

Legislation

9. Consideration should be given to the repeal of both the Surrogacy Arrangements Act 1985 and section 30 of the Human Fertilisation and Embryology Act 1990, and their replacement by a new Surrogacy Act. The Surrogacy Act would seek to address in the one statute the main legal principles governing surrogacy arrangements in the United Kingdom, to offer a surrogacy 'code' and include (paragraphs 7.2 and 7.3):

(i) the continuation of the current provisions of Section 1A of the 1985 Act relating to the non-enforceability of surrogacy contracts;

(ii) the continuation of current provisions prohibiting commercial agencies from assisting in the creation of surrogacy arrangements and related provisions prohibiting advertisements in relation to surrogacy arrangements;

(iii) new statutory provisions defining and limiting lawful payments to surrogate mothers;

(iv) provision for the promulgation by the UK Departments of Health of a Code of Practice governing surrogacy arrangements generally;

(v) provision for the registration of non profit-making surrogacy agencies by the Departments of Health and that such agencies should be required to comply with the Departments' Code of Practice on surrogacy arrangements;

(vi) provision to prohibit the operation of unregistered agencies;

(vii) new provisions for the grant of a parental order to commissioning couples (a revised section 30 order). The revised order should provide that applicants for a parental order should establish compliance with the Surrogacy Act and the Code of Practice; and that they have complied with the statutory limitations on payments. The revised order should *not* authorise the judge to approve otherwise impermissible payments.

10. Parental orders should only be obtained in the High Court; Judges should be able to order DNA tests; and Guardians *ad litem* should be able to check criminal records (paragraph 7.24).

11. In order for a parental order to be granted, the commissioning couple should be habitually resident in the United Kingdom, the Channel Islands or the Isle of Man for a period of 12 months immediately preceding the application for a parental order (paragraph 7.24).

Glossary of Terms Used **Annex A**

surrogacy Surrogacy is the practice whereby one woman (the *surrogate mother*) becomes pregnant, carries and gives birth to a child for another person(s) (*the commissioning couple*) as the result of an agreement prior to conception that the child should be handed over to that person after birth.

surrogate mother The woman who carries and gives birth to the child is the surrogate mother, or 'surrogate'. She may be the genetic mother ('partial' surrogacy) - *ie* using her own egg - or she may have an embryo - which may be provided by the *commissioning couple* - implanted in her womb using *in-vitro fertilisation (IVF) techniques* ('host' or 'full' surrogacy). Where the surrogacy is established using *in vitro fertilisation (IVF) or anonymous donor insemination*, this must (as with all uses of these techniques) take place in a clinic licensed by the Human Fertilisation and Embryology Authority (HFEA) under the terms of the Human Fertilisation and Embryology Act 1990. Such clinics are required to follow the provisions of the 1990 Act and the HFEA's Code of Practice, including a requirement to consider the welfare of any child born as a result of the treatment. Where IVF is not involved, the surrogate mother may attend a clinic to be inseminated or she may be inseminated artificially at home. If insemination occurs through sexual intercourse this may still constitute surrogacy.

commissioning couple The commissioning couple are the people who wish to bring up the child after his or her birth. They may both be the genetic parents, or one of them may be, or neither of them may be genetically related to the child. The woman for whom the child is to be carried (the 'commissioning mother') may be the genetic mother in that she provides the egg. The genetic father may be the husband or partner of the commissioning mother, or even of the carrying (surrogate) mother; or he may be an anonymous donor.

<u>Role of Guardians *ad litem*</u> **Annex B**

Introduction

Guardians *ad litem* and Reporting Officers (GALROs) are specialist social workers who act as officers of the court in family proceedings. There are about 850 GALROs in England and Wales; it is difficult to be precise because there is no national register and a proportion are members of more than one of the 54 English and 5 Welsh panels.

1. GALROs have two principal functions under the 1976 adoption legislation and a third role was introduced regarding parental orders with the implementation in 1994 of section 30 of the Human Fertilisation and Embryology Act 1990[44].

2. Under the Adoption Act 1976 there are two types of applications which involve GALROs. The first is for an adoption order (s 12) and the second a freeing order (s 18). Under the court rules of 1984 (as amended) a Guardian *ad litem* is appointed in an adoption application where the child has not been freed for adoption and it appears that the parent or guardian of the child is *un*willing to agree to the making of an adoption order. The duties of the Guardian *ad litem* are associated with safeguarding the interests of the child before the court. The rules require the Guardian to investigate the background leading to the application and any other relevant matter; to advise on whether the child should be present at the court hearing; to perform such other duties as appear to him or her as necessary or as the court may direct; and to prepare a confidential written report for the court.

3. The Reporting Officer is appointed in an adoption application where the child is not free for adoption and it appears that the parent or guardian *is* willing to agree to the making of an adoption order. The Reporting Officer's duties under the court rules are to ensure as far as is reasonably practicable that any agreement to the making of the adoption order is given freely and unconditionally and with a full understanding of what is involved; to witness the signature by the parent or guardian of the written agreement to the making of an adoption order; to investigate the circumstances relevant to that agreement; and to report in writing to the court drawing to the court's attention any matters which may assist the court in considering the application.

4. The respective roles of the Guardian *ad litem* and Reporting Officer in freeing applications are broadly similar to the above for adoption applications. A Guardian *ad litem* is appointed where the parent is unwilling to agree to the freeing application; a Reporting

---

44 See Local Authority Circular LAC(94)25 which provides detailed guidance on the powers and duties of Local Authorities, Health Authorities and Guardians *ad litem* under the terms of the Parental Orders (Human Fertilisation and Embryology) Regulations 1994

Officer is appointed where the parent prefers not to be involved in future questions concerning the adoption of the child and has made a declaration to that effect.

5. The role of the Guardian *ad litem* in section 30 parental orders is modelled on the earlier adoption court rules. Since section 30 orders cannot be made unless the surrogate mother agrees (section 30(5) of the 1990 Act), the focus of the Guardian *ad litem's* enquiries and written report to the court are on whether or not the requirements set out in section 30 are satisfied and whether there is any reason why the court should not make the parental order in the light of the child's welfare. There is no role for a reporting officer in the parental order provisions.

Summary of section 30 cases in England in which Guardians *ad litem* were involved (paragraphs 1.29-1.31)

No	Commissioning Couple			Surrogate Married/ Single	Expenses Paid £	Medical Oversight?
	Married/ Single	One or both genetically related?	Age: - Male - Female			
1	M	1	31-40 21-30	S	N/K	Y
2	M	1	31-40 31-40	S	620	N
3	M	1	31-40 48	M	3175	N
4	M	1	31-40 21-30	S	30	N
5	M	1	41+ 41+	M	0	N
6	M	BOTH	31-40 31-40	M	2730	Y
7	M	1	31-40 21-30	S	1177	N
8	M	1	31-40 31-40	S	5250	N
9	M	1	31-40 31-40	S	8000	N
10	M	1	31-40 31-40	M	12000	N
11	M	1	21-30 21-30	M	2000	N
12	M	BOTH	31-40 21-30	M	5124	Y
13	M	1	31-40 31-40	S	2000	N
14	M	1	31-40 31-40	S	100	N
15	M	1	41+ 41+	M	0	N
16	M	1	41+ 31-40	S	2028	N

No	Commissioning Couple			Surrogate Married/ Single	Expenses Paid £	Medical Oversight?
	Married/ Single	One or both genetically related?	Age: - Male - Female			
17	M	BOTH	31-40 31-40	M	0	Y
18	M	BOTH	31-40 21-30	M	4021	Y
19	M	1	31-40 -	M	5720	N
20	M	1	41+ 31-40	M	3200	N
21	M	1	41+ 31-40	S	1800	N
22	M	1	31-40 31-40	S	8000	Y
23	M	BOTH	41+ 31-40	M	1200	Y
24	M	1	31-40 31-40	M	9275	N
25	M	BOTH	31-40 31-40	M	4660	Y
26	M	BOTH	31-40 31-40	S	8651	Y
27	M	1	31-40 31-40	S	1000	N
28	M	1	31-40 31-40	S	8000	N
29	M	1	31-40 31-40	S	2321	N
30	M	BOTH	- -	S	700	Y
31	M	1	41+ 41+	M	1600	N
32	M	1	41+ 41+	S	5600	N
33	M	1	31-40 31-40	M	1000	N
34	M	1	31-40 31-40	M	N/K	Y

total number of children involved = 39

Questions asked in the public consultation document **Annex D**

Q1. Should there be a legal ban on all payments to the surrogate mother made by or on behalf of the commissioning parents?

Q2. If payments could be made:

i. should this include remuneration by way of payment for carrying the child;

ii. should it include reimbursement for loss of actual earnings;

iii. should it include compensation for loss of potential earnings (*ie* where the surrogate mother was not actually in work at the time the arrangements are made);

iv. should it include only relevant expenses (*ie* those expenses which can be directly related to the cost of bearing the child *eg* maternity clothing, travel expenses etc) incurred in the pregnancy?

Q3. If remuneration and/or relevant expenses could be paid, should there be legislation to define what can be included?

Q4. If your answer to Q3 is 'yes:

i. what should relevant expenses include?

ii. should there be a maximum payable?

- for remuneration?

- for expenses?

Q5. Should there be a body to regulate and/or monitor surrogacy arrangements?

i. if established, should the body also regulate and/or monitor surrogacy agencies?

ii. do you have any views on the kind of regulatory body it should be, or the expertise required for it to function? are there any existing bodies which provide a model?

Q6. Should the law:

i. allow agencies to continue on their current, informal, basis?

ii. restrict their operation further (possibly including a total ban)?

iii. put them on a more formal footing?

Q7. If agencies are to be involved in making surrogacy arrangements should they have to be approved?

Q8. If agencies were to make surrogacy arrangements, should couples be free to decide whether to use the services of an agency or not?

Public consultation: statistical summary of all responses. **Annex E1**

Number of responses = 369

	number who responded to the question	Answered Yes		Answered No	
Should there be a legal ban on all payments to the surrogate mother made by or on behalf of the commissioning parents ?	349	39	11.17%	310	88.83%
Should payments include remuneration by way of payment for carrying the child?	338	202	59.76%	136	40.24%
Should it include remuneration for loss of actual earnings?	337	277	82.20%	60	17.80%
Should it include reimbursement for loss of potential earnings ?	330	157	47.58%	173	52.42%
Should it include only relevant expenses incurred in the pregnancy ?	325	156	48.00%	169	52.00%
If remuneration and/or relevant expenses could be paid,should there be legislation to define what can be included ?	331	266	80.36%	65	18.62%
Should there be a maximum payable for remuneration?	260	207	79.62%	53	20.38%
Should there be maximum payable for expenses ?	265	206	77.74%	59	22.26%
Should there be a body to regulate and /or monitor surrogacy arrangements ?	331	287	86.71%	44	13.29%
Should there be a body to regulate and/or monitor surrogacy agencies ?	329	147	93.01%	23	6.99%
Should the law allow agencies to continue on their current, informal basis?	328	71	44.82%	181	55.18%
Should the law restrict their operation further (possibly including a total ban) ?	326	71	21.78%	255	78.22%
Should the law put agencies on a more formal footing?	321	278	86.60%	43	13.40%
If agencies are to be involved in making surrogacy arrangements should they have to be approved ?	328	307	93.60%	21	6.40%
If agencies were to make surrogacy arrangements should couples be free to decide whether to use the services of an agency or not ?	315	239	75.87%	76	24.13%

<u>Public consultation</u>: responses <u>excluding</u> COTS' members. **Annex E2**

Number of responses = 247

	number who responded to the question	Answered Yes		Answered No	
Should there be a legal ban on all payments to the surrogate mother made by or on behalf of the commissioning parents ?	227	38	16.74%	189	83.26%
Should payments include remuneration by way of payment for carrying the child?	221	97	43.89%	124	56.11%
Should it include remuneration for loss of actual earnings?	219	164	74.89%	55	25.11%
Should it include reimbursement for loss of potential earnings ?	216	68	31.48%	148	68.52%
Should it include only relevant expenses incurred in the pregnancy ?	208	116	55.77%	92	44.23%
If remuneration and/or relevant expenses could be paid,should there be legislation to define what can be included ?	216	167	77.31%	49	21.59%
Should there be a maximum payable for remuneration?	158	112	70.89%	46	29.11%
Should there be maximum payable for expenses ?	168	123	73.21%	45	26.79%
Should there be a body to regulate and /or monitor surrogacy arrangements ?	218	195	89.45%	23	10.55%
Should there be a body to regulate and/or monitor surrogacy agencies ?	215	199	92.56%	16	7.44%
Should the law allow agencies to continue on their current, informal basis?	217	53	24.42%	164	75.58%
Should the law restrict their operation further (possibly including a total ban)?	206	68	33.01%	138	66.99%
Should the law put agencies on a more formal footing?	212	181	85.38%	31	14.62%
If agencies are to be involved in making surrogacy arrangements should they have to be approved ?	215	201	93.49%	14	6.51%
If agencies were to make surrogacy arrangements should couples be free to decide whether to use the services of an agency or not ?	202	133	65.84%	69	34.16%

List of those who provided oral evidence to the review **Annex F**

Austin, Clare
Surrogacy Parenting Centre

Baker, Miranda Ms
Hinchliffe, Michael Mr
Solicitors' Family Law Association

Brinsden, Peter Dr
British Fertility Society

Burchell, David Mr
Speirs, Jennifer Ms
Blyth, Eric Mr
British Association of Social Workers

Cotton, Kim Ms
Baldwin, Mark Mr
Childlessness Overcome Through Surrogacy

Deech, Ruth Mrs
McCarthy, Suzanne Mrs
Heales, Beatrice Ms
Human Fertilisation and Embryology Authority

Hunt, Jennifer Ms
Blyth, Eric Mr
British Infertility Counselling Association

Richards, Jim Mr
Timms, Judith Ms
Catholic Child Welfare Council

Wilks, Michael Dr
Morgan, Derek Mr
Sommerville, Ann Ms
British Medical Association

Wilson-Thomas, Claire Mrs
Taylor, Phillipa Ms
Christian Action Research and Education

Other individuals who gave evidence wished to remain anonymous

<u>List of those who attended the seminar on 6 April 1998</u> (see para 1.46) Annex G

Professor Margaret Brazier	Professor of Law, University of Manchester; Chairman of surrogacy review committee
Professor Alastair Campbell	Professor of Ethics in Medicine, University of Bristol; member of surrogacy review committee
Professor Susan Golombok	Professor of Psychology, City University London; member of surrogacy review committee
Mr Michael Evans	Department of Health; secretary to the surrogacy review
Dr Kenneth Boyd	Institute of Medical Ethics, University of Edinburgh
Dr Heather Draper	Centre for Biomedical Ethics, University of Birmingham
Dr Gavin Fairbairn	Reader in Education/Social Work, North East Wales Institute
Mrs Marcia Fry	Branch Head, Department of Health
Dr Elaine Gadd	Senior Medical Officer, Department of Health
The Hon Mrs Justice Hale	High Court Judge
Mrs Kerry Herivel	Guardian *ad litem*, West Sussex
Dr Maggie Kirk	School of Nursing and Midwifery, University of Glamorgan
Mr Tony McGleenan	School of Law, Queen's University, Belfast
Professor J K Mason	Faculty of Law, University of Edinburgh
Mr Derek Morgan	Cardiff Law School and member BMA medical ethics committee
Rev'd Dr John Polkinghorne	Chairman Science, Medicine and Technology Committee, Board of Social Responsibility General Synod of the Church of England
Mrs Judith Timms	Chief Executive, National Youth Advocacy Service

List of respondents to the consultation document[45] Annex H

Akker, Dr O. van den

Alberti, K.G.M.M.
Royal College Of Physicians.

Allinson,M.

Anderson, C.

Andrean Mrs. R.M.

Ashcroft, Dr. Richard.
McNeill, Professor Paul.
Centre for Ethics In Medicine, University of Bristol.

Atkin, Jane.

Baker, Miranda.
Hinchliffe, Mike.
SFLA Children Committee.

Balen, Dr. Adam H.
Leeds General Infirmary.

Barley, Jeremy.
Association of Lawyers for Children.

Barnes, P.

Barnes, Dame Josephine.

Baron, Professor D.N.

Begley, Ann. M.
School Of Nursing and Midwifery, The Queens University of Belfast.

Bekir, J.S.
London Women's Clinic.

Bennett, Kate.

Bernard, Lulu.

Birmingham Women's Hospital

Black, D.J.
University Of Glamorgan.

Blake, Mr. J.

Blyth, Eric.
Social Work, University of Huddersfield.

Bolton, Dr. L.M.
Ysbyty Gwynedd, Wales.

Booth, Sheila.
Merthyr Tydfil Social Services Dept.

Booth, Penelope J.
University of Teeside.

Bowden, S.

Boyle, Dr. David.
Regional Fertility Clinic, Belfast.

Brannigan, Tracy.

Brazendale, J.

Brinsden, Peter.
Medical Director, Bourn Hall Clinic.

Brown, Mrs, A.M.

Brown, Clare.
Executive Director, CHILD.

Brunner-Ellis, Anne & Robin.

Bunce, T.J & L.L.

Callman, Judy.

Campbell, A.S.
Royal College of Surgeons of Glasgow.

CARE at The Park Hospital, Centre for Assisted Reproduction.

Carr, Katherine Elizabeth.

Carter, Robin.

Clinical And Scientific Committee, Family Planning and Reproductive Health Care, Royal College of Obstetricians and Gynaecologists.

Codling, Sally-Anne.

Cohen, Rowena.
Cardiff Community Healthcare.

Colchester, Charlie.
Christian Action, Research and Education. (CARE)

Collins, Ms L.J.

Conway, David.

Cotton, G & K.

Covell, J.

Cox, John & Sarah.

Creasey, M.

Cunningham, B.

Davies, Ruth.

Davies, David.

Davies, Mr & Mrs. M.D.

Davis, Patricia.

Dawson, K.J.

Deech, Ruth.
Human Fertilisation and Embryology Authority.

Deffenze, Susanne.
Health Visitor, Royal Alexandra Hospital, Rhyl.

Dickenson, Dr Donna L.
Imperial College.

Dodd, John.

Dodd, Gena.
COTS

Donaldson, Mrs F.

Draper, Dr. Heather.
Centre for Biomedical Ethics, University of Birmingham.

Dyker, Dr. George S.
Royal College of General Practitioners, Scottish Council.

Easton, David.
The Church of Scotland.

Elstein, Professor Max.

Emery, Simon.
Singleton Hospital.

Entwhistle, Paul.

---

45 There were 369 responses. 281 were marked non-confidential, though some of these were submitted anonymously; 79 were marked confidential and 9 partially confidential - see paragraphs 1.36-1.40. This is a list only of those marked non-confidential which included the name of the respondent(s).

Ferguson, Polly.
The Royal College Of Midwives, Welsh Board.

Field, Jane.

Field, A.M.

Fischer, Jana E.

Foreman, Robert.
Centre For Reproductive Medicine.

Frankland, Jayne & Mark.

Fraser, Rev. Andrew.
Free Church Of Scotland.

Gartlan, Jenny.
U.N.D.A.H. Trust, Belfast.

Giesen, Julie, A.

Gillies, L.
St. Columba's Church Of Scotland.

Gladwin, Martin.
Devon Panel Of Guardians *ad litem* and Reporting Officers.

Green, T

Griffiths, Mary.
British Association Of Social Workers, Scotland.

Hall, K.

Hancock, Christine.
Royal College of Nursing.

Harding, Dr. J. R.
Royal Gwent Hospital.

Harpwood, Vivienne.
Cardiff Law School.

Harris, John
University of Manchester

Hartnoll, Mary, C.
Social Work, Glasgow City Council.

Hartshorne,Susan.
Infertility Services and Ethical Committee. St. Mary's Hospital, Manchester.

Hazell, Suzanne.
School Of Nursing Studies, University Hospital Of Wales.

Healey, Maria.

Herivel, Mrs.
West Sussex Panel of Guardians *ad litem* and Reporting Officers.

Hickey, Mrs. S.

Hinds, Mary.
Hillman, Joe.
Nursing Officers, DHSS (NI)

Hogewind, Dr. George.
London Gynaecology and Fertility Centre.

Holmes-Siedle, Dr. Monica.

Holt, Nicola.

Hope, Tony.
Institute Of Health Sciences, Oxford.

Howe, Kerrie.
Supervisor for Infertility Counselling, Ninewells Hospital, Dundee.

Howells, Debbie.

Howie, Professor P.W.
University of Dundee.

Inglis, Dr Sheila M.C.
Children In Scotland.

Jackson, Megan.

Johns, Peter.
North Gwent Community Health Council.

Johnson and Dawson Drs
A.C.V. Chelsea and Westminster Hospital.

Jones, Pat.
University of Huddersfield.

Jones, Sandy.

Jones, Dr. M.W.

Joyce, Dr.D.
Director, Fertility Services, Southmead Hospital, Bristol.

Kennedy, Richard,
Director, Centre For Reproductive Medicine, Coventry.

Kenyon, Penny.

Kerr, Janice.

Killick, Professor S.
Director, Hull IVF Unit.

Kimber, S.

Kirton, Ian.

Klewis, Miss.

Knowles, Amanda.

Lawrence, Nick.
Social Services Dept. Ebbw Vale, Gwent.

Lowe, M.J.
British Medical Association.

Lowe, Alison.
Leeds City Council Women's Committee.

MacDermot, Jean.

MacIntosh, Calum.

MacKenzie, Lorna.

Mackinnon, Judith.

Macnaughton, Professor Sir Malcolm.

Mahon, Hilda & Dean.

Marshall, Neil.
General Medical Council.

Martin, P.K.

Martin, Dr. D.H.
Altnagalvin Hospital, Londonderry.

Mason, Professor, J.K.
University of Edinburgh.

Masson, Gordon M.
Chalybeate Hospital, Hampshire.

Matthews, Professor Eric.
University Of Aberdeen.

McDowall, Colin.

McDowall, Margaret.

McCaughey, G.

McEwan, Leslie.
Social Work, City of Edinburgh Council.

McGinnis, E.B.
MENCAP.

McLean, Professor Sheila A.M.
University of Glasgow.

McNaught, Pamela & Murray.

McWhinnie, Alexina.
Social Work, University of Dundee.

Mead, Professor Donna.
School of Nursing and Midwifery, University of Glamorgan.

Mendez, M & C.

Midwifery Lecturers at the School of Nursing and Midwifery, University of Wales, Bangor.

Miles, Marjorie.

Mills, John.
Ninewells Hospital and Medical School, Dundee.

Milne, Miss Helen.

Mitchell, Mr. & Mrs. B.

Molony, Pauline.
The Patients' Association.

Monahan, Julie.

Morgan, T.

O'Brien, Mr & Mrs R.

Parsons,Andrew.
Radcliffes Solicitors.

Patel, Sir Naren.
Royal College of Obstetricians and Gynaecologists.

Paterson, S.

Pearce, Amanda.

Perks, Nigel F.
The Fertility Centre, St. Bartholomew's Hospital.

Phipps, Rev, Terence E.
Guild Of Catholic Doctors.

Potter, Dr. Brian T.
British Medical Association, Scotland.

Price, A.E.

Price, David. P.T.
School of Law, De Montfort University.

Revd. Dr. John Polkinghorne.
Science, Medicine and Technology Committee, Church of England.

Rice, Susan.
The National Fertility Association.

Richards, J.M.
Catholic Child Welfare Council.

Hon. Lady Roache J.P.
Ethics Committee, Cromwell Hospital.

Roberts, Dr Jeremy A.

Robertson, W.B.
Social Worker, Angus Council.

Robinson, Linda.

Rodger, Dr. J.
Royal College of General Practitioners.

Salvetti, Roger.
Biscoe, Cousins, Groves Solicitors.

Saunders, Dr. John.
Neville Hall Hospital, Gwent.

Sharples, F.W.

Shawyer, Neil & Kim.

Skinnner, Adrian.

Slevin, Professor O D'A.
National Board For Nursing, Midwifery and Health Visiting.

Smith, Jacqueline.

Smyth, W. Martin. (MP)

Soathon, Meg.
Neath General Hospital, Wales.

Steene, Jill.
United Kingdom Central Council for Nursing, Midwifery and Health Visiting.

Stevenson, D.M.

Stewart, Dr. Margaret.
County Durham Health Authority.

Stone, Julie.
Centre For Biomedical Ethics, University of Birmingham.

Sutton, Agneta.
Centre For Bioethics and Public Policy.

Theodore,A.
Royal College Of Nursing.

Thomas, J. St.J.
Royal College Of Physicians, Scotland.

Thomas, Rosamund.
Vale of Glamorgan Community Health Council.

Thomas-Peter, K.M.

Town, J.S. & C.A.

Van Meeuwen, Anne.
Barnardos.

Walker, R & J.

Walton, Wendy.

Walton. P.
Cheshire Guardian *ad litem* and Reporting Officer Panel.

Whipp, Christine.

Williams, Mrs C.

Williams, Dan R.
Carmarthen/Dinefwr Community Health Council.

Williamson, Jayne.
University of Aberdeen.

Windsor, Mrs. J.

Winter, R.
Secretary, Association of Directors of Social Work, Scotland.

Wood, Mrs Christina.

Wright, Amanda.

Wyatt, Irene F.

Printed in the UK for The Stationery Office Limited on behalf of the
Controller of Her Majesty's Stationery Office
Dd 5068361 10/98 61743 Job No 62022